First Step for
NCLEX-PN
SUCCESS

First Step for
NCLEX-PN
SUCCESS

Donald L. Anderson, RN, EdD

Assistant Professor
Regis College
Weston, Massachusetts
Director, Test Preparation Specialists, Inc.
Billerica, Massachusetts

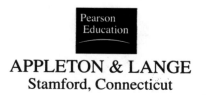

Pearson
Education

APPLETON & LANGE
Stamford, Connecticut

Pearson
Education

Copyright © 1998 by Appleton & Lange
A Simon & Schuster Company

All rights reserved. This book, or any parts thereof, may not be used or reproduced in any manner without written permission. For information, address Appleton & Lange, 107 Elm Street, P.O. Box 120041, Stamford, CT 06912-0041.

www.appletonlange.com

PN Success is a registered trademark of the Arnett Development Corporation for NCLEX-PN computer adaptive software. For further information on this product, please contact Arnett Development Corporation, PO Box 6326, North Augusta, SC 29861. (803) 279-6325

98 99 00 00 01 02 / 10 9 8 7 6 5 4 3 2 1

Prentice Hall International (UK) Limited, London
Prentice Hall of Australia Pty. Limited, Sydney
Prentice Hall Canada, Inc., Toronto
Prentice Hall Hispanoamericana, S.A., Mexico
Prentice Hall of India Private Limited, New Delhi
Prentice Hall of Japan, Inc., Tokyo
Simon and Schuster Asia Pte. Ltd., Singapore
Editora Prentice Hall do Brasil Ltda., Rio de Janeiro
Prentice Hall, Upper Saddle River, New Jersey

Library of Congress Catalog Card Number: 97-077501

ISBN 0-8385-2601-2

90000

9 780838 526019

Acquisitions Editor: David P. Carroll
Production Editor: Sondra Greenfield
Production Services: Rainbow Graphics, Inc.
Designer: Janice Barsevich Bielawa

PRINTED IN THE UNITED STATES OF AMERICA

Dedication

To the families of nursing graduates
for their sacrifice and support of their loved ones.

To the faculty members of nursing programs
who commit their time, effort, and energy in preparing
students to become the best nurses they can be.

Contents

Preface

Nursing school curricula are designed to educate students to provide safe and appropriate patient care. This book has been developed to assist practical and vocational nursing students to focus their studying on information that they are likely to encounter when taking the NCLEX-PN examination. The licensing examination is the final hurdle encountered prior to practicing as a licensed vocational/practical nurse. The National Council of State Boards of Nursing, Inc. has been charged with developing and administering the nursing licensing examination. Graduate nurses' knowledge of nursing is demonstrated on the NCLEX-PN CAT, utilizing a multiple-choice format. Successful completion of this examination heralds entry of the graduate nurse into the world of practical nursing.

Understanding "the rules of the game" (or in this case, the rules of the test) will assist the graduate nurse in understanding how the examination is structured and the way the questions are developed. This essential information will assist you in developing your study plan for the boards. Understanding the rules will allow you to take control of the examination, rather than letting it control you. Part One of this book offers a description of the NCLEX-PN examination design. It provides information related to the structure and format of the test and the organization of the questions. This portion of the book also supplies the framework of a study plan of attack that includes the development of an understanding of the multiple-choice question format. This section is full of test-taking strategies that you can use to improve your performance on the boards. These strategies allow the test taker a way to narrow down correct answers and improve their testing performance. A relaxation technique is presented that can assist in lowering anxiety levels during examinations. If you are the type of person who has difficulty taking a multiple-choice examination, this section is essential to study and integrate into your test-taking practice.

Parts 2-, 3-, and 4 of this book are devoted to offering information that is important to know when preparing for the NCLEX-PN CAT. Part 2 is developed on a systems approach format that incorporates essential facts, safety tips, and points to ponder. This section covers adult health and is developed from a number of sources, including faculty members teaching various specialty areas, students, graduate nurses, and the author's analysis of important areas identified by the National Council itself as part of job performance studies.

Part 3 isolates specific specialty areas and the high probability of testing areas associated with these. This section includes information about pediatric nursing, psychosocial issues and nursing care, communication techniques, and gerontologic points of importance.

Part 4 of this book contains pharmacologic information. It includes a group of commonly used categories of medications, the indications for use, side effects, and the nursing implications of each medication or category. All three sections focus on *high index of probability items* (HIP items) and information that will assist you in your studying. These sections are not meant to be a comprehensive area of study; rather, the purpose of these sections is to help the graduate to distinguish the "need to know" material from the nonessential information, or the "nice to know" material, which is not likely to be tested on this NCLEX-PN CAT.

Part 5 of the book presents a list and description of various NCLEX-PN review books written to assist you in preparing for the examination. The NCLEX-PN books are divided into two categories. A comprehensive review book is designed to provide a synopsis of all the information covered in your nursing program. Some of these books may also include multiple-choice questions, answers, and rationales for the answers. The other type of book described is referred to as a Q&A or question and answer book. These books contain some information on testing followed by a large number of questions and answers, including rationales for the responses. Comments written in this section are provided by graduate nurses, who have already taken the NCLEX-PN and have spent time reviewing the books, based on their opinions and experiences.

Part 6, the final section in the book, is a 205-item examination designed to test your knowledge in high-index or high-probability items. The examination has a multiple-choice question format similar to the NCLEX-PN exam and includes four options. The rationales for each correct and incorrect response have been developed to assist the tester in understanding why answers are correct and incorrect. The rationales have been validated for correctness by using standard nursing texts. A computer disk that includes this same information is also supplied for the book, so you can take the test on computer in either a testing format or a tutorial format.

Graduate nurses, students, and faculty members are encouraged to submit ideas, testing tips, mnemonics, and suggestions to assist their future colleagues in studying for the NCLEX-PN CAT. We are also interested in your opinions of the NCLEX-PN CAT study books you use and what you feel the strengths and weaknesses of the books are. Please see the section on how to contribute to send us your comments and ideas. *A word of caution:* We are not interested in information about your specific examination. The sharing of questions and answers from the NCLEX-PN CAT examination is prohibited and considered an unethical practice for nurses. The purpose of this book is to provide you with a way to share your experiences and ideas on how to study for examinations and ways to retain the information. Please spend a few minutes filling out the contributor form, and you will be rewarded with a discount coupon for another Appleton & Lange publication of your choice.

We wish you good luck and good testing!

Acknowledgments

Nursing is a demanding and giving profession. It is a special type of people who spend their time improving the health of others. In these busy times, it can be difficult to devote additional help to future colleagues. I gratefully acknowledge future graduate nurses for their contribution to this project. By spending time assisting their peers, they offer some of themselves and their wisdom in becoming successful on the examination. I would like to acknowledge the following individuals for their special efforts and thoughts on this edition: Anthony Brodeur, Gil Burden, Jennifer Bourassa, Heather Burr, Dawn Carman, Jason Corriveau, John Coy, Dawn Dangora, Dianne Hamilton-Toles, Guv Impietro, Paul Jodrey, John Johnson, Everett Kennision, Jr., Monique Laflamme, Barbara Meng, Terry Nordmann, Marc Nordstrom, Nerine O'Neil, Jodrey Paul, John Pina, Barbara Quenneville, Marc Therian, Joseph Thompson, Philip Verzani, and James Weston. These individuals were essential by providing ideas and comments.

Our families have been supportive throughout this project, and I especially acknowledge my loving wife, Joanne, and loving sons, Jason and Ryan, for their continued encouragement throughout this and other projects.

I would also like to thank three key people at Appleton & Lange who have continued to encourage me throughout the project: Sally Barhydt, Dave Carroll, and Sondra Greenfield. Their contributions, suggestions, and ideas have been instrumental in bringing this project forward. Their knowledge and professionalism allow authors to produce their best efforts in providing the graduate nurse with important information necessary to prepare for the NCLEX-PN. Finally, a word of thanks to the staff of Rainbow Graphics for their able assistance on this project. Their tolerance for changes and "making it right" is unsurpassed.

Thank you all.

Donald L. Anderson, RN, EdD

Contributors

Barbara Ahern, RN, MSN
Director of Practical Nursing
Shawsheen Valley Regional Technical High School
  and School of Practical Nursing
Billerica, Massachusetts

CPT Patricia Brigham, RN, MEd, CNA
OIC/NCLEX-PN Review Program
U.S. Army Reserve
Regis College
Weston, Massachusetts

LTC Linda S. Goodale, RN, MSN
OIC RN/BSN Completion Program
U.S. Army Reserve
Regis College
Weston, Massachusetts

Patricia Noonan, RN, BSN
Instructor
Shawsheen Valley Regional Technical High School
  and School of Practical Nursing
Billerica, Massachusetts

Linda Tenofsky, RNC, PhD
Associate Professor
Division of Nursing Studies
Curry College
Milton, Massachusetts

How to Contribute

It is our intent to use this book as a forum for graduating nurses, student nurses, nursing faculty, and nursing staff. We encourage everyone to submit their ideas for inclusion in this book and hope it becomes viewed as a vehicle to disseminate information and ways to be better prepared for the NCLEX-PN CAT.

We encourage you to submit any suggestions you have by providing

- Additional facts, mnemonics, and test-taking strategies proven to help you understand complex areas.
- Other information you feel may be helpful and of benefit to your colleagues.
- Personal ratings and reviews/comments about the review books, computer disks, and other study material you have used in preparation for the NCLEX-PN CAT. See the rating scale at the beginning of Part 5.

NOTE TO CONTRIBUTORS

With the advent of computerized adaptive examinations, individuals will receive a test that is unique to them, created from a question bank of hundreds and thousands of items. We do not encourage individuals to submit any information pertaining to their own examination, especially information about individual questions. We refer you to the ethical commitment described by the National Council of State Boards of Nursing, Inc., which precludes "unauthorized possession, reproduction, or disclosure of the nature or content of examination questions, before, during, or after the examination as it is in violation of the law." In addition, conveying this information is considered an unethical practice for professionals, which we discourage. Rather, we ask that you include information you have gathered during your studies as a nursing student and in your review as a graduate nurse preparing for the NCLEX-PN CAT.

You can mail typed entries or computer disks (Microsoft Works) to: *First Step for NCLEX-PN Success,* Appleton & Lange, 107 Elm Street, P.O. Box 120041, Stamford, CT 06912-0041 (Attention: Contributions). You will be recognized by a letter from the author, which will document your addition to this book if it is used. This letter can be used by you in your annual performance reviews as evidence of your participation in professional activities. We reserve the right to edit and review the material that has been submitted for inclusion in this book. No material will be returned.

Contributions for High Index of Probability Items
(Parts 2, 3, and 4)

Name of Contributor _____

Affiliation or School _____

Address _____

_____

Telephone Number _____

Section:

Fact to Be Included:

Section:

Fact to Be Included:

Section:

Fact to Be Included:

Section:

Fact to Be Included:

Section:

Fact to Be Included:

You will receive a personal acknowledgment and a $10 coupon toward selected Appleton & Lange books for material that is used in future editions.

- (fold here) -

Return Address

_____

_____

_____

Postage
required

Attn: Contributions
First Step for NCLEX-PN Success
Appleton & Lange
107 Elm Street, P.O. Box 120041
Stamford, CT 06912-0041

- (fold here) -

Contributions for Book Reviews (Part 5)

Name of Contributor _____

Affiliation or School _____

Address _____

_____

Telephone Number _____

Author and Title:

Edition: _____ Publication Year: _____ Rating: _____ Publisher: _____ ISBN: _____

Strengths: _____

_____

_____

_____

Weaknesses: _____

_____

_____

_____

Author and Title:

Edition: _____ Publication Year: _____ Rating: _____ Publisher: _____ ISBN: _____

Strengths: _____

_____

_____

_____

Weaknesses: _____

_____

_____

_____

Author and Title:

Edition: _____ Publication Year: _____ Rating: _____ Publisher: _____ ISBN: _____

Strengths: _____

_____

_____

_____

Weaknesses: _____

_____

_____

_____

You will receive a personal acknowledgment and a $10 coupon toward selected Appleton & Lange books for material that is used in future editions.

User Survey

Name of Contributor _____

Affiliation or School _____

Address _____

_____

Telephone Number _____

What advice would you give a student or graduating nurse preparing for the NCLEX-PN CAT?

What did you like most or least about this book? Do you have any suggestions for ways in which it might be improved?

Do you have any suggestions for the test-taking strategies in Part 1?

Were there any high index of probability items in Parts 2, 3, or 4 that you feel are unnecessary and should be deleted? (To suggest items that should be included, please use the separate form.)

You will receive a personal acknowledgment and a $10 coupon toward selected Appleton & Lange books for material that is used in future editions.

--(fold here)--

Return Address

_____

_____

_____

Postage
required

Attn: Contributions
First Step for NCLEX-PN Success
Appleton & Lange
107 Elm Street, P.O. Box 120041
Stamford, CT 06912-0041

--(fold here)--

PART I

▶ Prepare Smart: Test Smart

- Introduction
- What the NCLEX-PN CAT Is
- Success Rate for the NCLEX-PN CAT
- Categories of Testing for the NCLEX-PN CAT
- Taking the NCLEX-PN CAT Examination
- Registering and Taking the NCLEX-PN CAT
- Rumors, Rantings, and Ravings
- Manage and Conquer Your Test-taking Anxiety
- Test for Success: Passing the Examination
- Strategies for Taking the NCLEX-PN CAT
- What to Expect After the Exam

INTRODUCTION

You are finishing your nursing education, getting ready to graduate, and everyone is congratulating you and asking questions like "What will you do now?" or "Do you have a job yet?" or "Where are you going to work?" Feeling a sense of relief at finishing school, you still experience a twinge of uneasiness because unlike other school programs, your days of studying are not yet finished. The discomfort you feel is natural, experienced by many graduates, and is justified because you have one more (very large) hoop to jump through or hurdle to get over. The dreaded "State Board Exam," officially known as the National Council Licensure Examination for Practical Nurses Computer Adaptive Test (NCLEX-PN CAT), looms on the horizon. Graduation parties are fun, but few family and friends recognize the additional burden on your shoulders to become a *licensed* practical/vocational nurse.

Are You One of These Types ▶ of Graduates?

How you respond to this challenge depends on how you have responded to challenges in the past. Different backgrounds and experiences all help to mold our personalities. There are an infinite number of ways to respond to this test, and over the years I have seen a number of "test-taking" personalities including the Lethargic Doubter, the Procrastinator, the Anxious Fatalist, the Go-Getter, the Super-Organizer, and the Attacker.

The Lethargic Doubter

Lethargic Doubters experience a "letdown" upon program completion because they feel as though they have put all of the energy they possess into their student learning. They have great difficulty summoning up the energy to "gear up" for another round of late-night studying and reviewing information they learned once already. They can be heard to say, "I don't have the time to study for this examination. I need to make money now, so I will worry about the examination later." Lethargic Doubters promptly fall asleep every time they open any type of a review book. They will take the examination with little or no preparation and may develop a fear of failure even before they arrive at the test center.

The Procrastinator

Procrastinators can fill in the blank of "I will study . . . tomorrow . . . next week . . . next month . . . next year . . . or . . . the day before the examination." They deny the reality of taking the NCLEX-PN CAT and put it off or avoid study whenever possible. When they eventually sit down to review material, they will soon begin to look around and see a dirty rug, a sinkful of dishes, a dusty coffee table, or a dirty bathroom. After sitting in front of the book for several more minutes, they have an intense urge to clean the area that they have identified as being filthy. Cleaning becomes the priority and it can't wait any longer (they justify), so after 10 full minutes of intense study, they begin vigorous cleaning for the rest of the day. They have the best intentions the next day but again talk themselves out of reviewing by adding additional tasks to their priority list (like food shopping, holiday shopping, or going to the gym). Rationalizing their approach, Procrastinators say, "You can't really study for the NCLEX-PN CAT anyway, so I might as well not put too much effort into study." The Procrastinator enters the test site with a good dose of guilt and a small amount of confidence.

The Anxious Fatalist

Anxious Fatalists rush out to buy every piece of material ever produced to study for the NCLEX-PN CAT. Their anxiety is heightened when they talk to other friends/colleagues who are preparing with materials they don't own. They live in fear that they are not studying the right information and believe that they must study 12 to 18 hours per day for 3 months and 4$\frac{1}{2}$ days. Sitting and relaxing without doing something makes them very anxious, and they feel comfortable only with a book constantly in their hand. Anxious Fatalists work and work and work to the point of burnout, and focus on what they don't know rather than what they know and have learned. In spite of all the effort invested, they maintain an attitude of "I've never tested well, so I probably won't pass this test anyway." Anxious Fatalists enter the test center with a very high level of anxiety.

The Go-Getter

Every school has at least one (or more) of these people. They seem ever confident and ready to take charge of any situation. They have an aura about them which conveys success. Go-Getters are risk takers who are able to control their anxiety. They are very adaptable and move from the student role to the graduate nurse role with ease. Go-Getters are people who have job offers before graduation when most students are still thinking about what is due in the morning. Go-Getters have boundless energy for study in spite of a busy schedule. They always seem to get twice as much done as anyone else, and always seem to maintain a positive attitude. They enter the examination confident and with a feeling of anticipation.

The Organizer

Organizers set specific goals and lay out plans to accomplish them. They are living "the nursing process" and look at everything in terms of how to break down tasks into specific pieces. Organizers are known for developing study patterns such as using multiple color-coded pads of paper or note cards, using several different colors of ink to take notes, and frequently recopying lecture notes immediately after class. They keep different calendars for each part of their life, may actually carry more than one around, and feel particularly anxious unless they are totally organized. They function very well when they can organize their day. Organizers arrive at the center one hour prior to their appointment to avoid being late. They are usually confident if they can maintain their structure or routine.

The Attacker

Attackers take the bull by the horns but can sometimes go off misdirected. These people look at life events as a competition and in win–lose terms. When they develop an effective study plan, they can accomplish a great deal, but without a firm plan, they can get into trouble. Attackers are sometimes considered flighty or unpredictable and may sometimes be labeled as troublemakers. They may look at the NCLEX-PN CAT as a competition and can get sidetracked fighting a battle on why they have to take the examination as opposed to how to study for this examination. When they get into a fighting mode, they can waste a lot of their energy spinning their wheels in futile causes. When they are put on the right track, they can be highly successful. They usually enter the test site prepared and ready, but must take care to control their anger.

Do you recognize anyone? To be sure, this is an obvious oversimplification of test-taking personalities, but many might recognize parts of themselves among these categories. Although they are described in a tongue-in-cheek fashion, there is one commonality that all of these personalities (and anyone else) who are taking a comprehensive entry-level practice examination will require: They must develop an organized approach to reviewing nursing information that will yield the greatest amount of pertinent data in the least (reasonable) amount of time. A plan helps reduce anxiety to overcome the initial *period of panic,* which is characterized by a feeling of impending doom and being completely overwhelmed. This panic can paralyze test takers and prevent them from studying effectively for the NCLEX-PN CAT. The hours spent in the panic period generate a tremendous amount of "needless" or "useless" energy and can be counterproductive to good preparation.

The panic period is normal and expected. However, the person must take control over the situation, recognize this initial high level of anxiety, and develop a plan of study that will work for them. Any plan created must be NCLEX-PN directed. Unfortunately, many graduate nurses lack an understanding of this and begin by studying every lecture note they ever took during nursing school. In addition, they may fail to properly allocate their study time to yield the most productive results, and this ineffectiveness usually proves to be counterproductive to their success.

Development of an effective plan involves obtaining a clear picture of what the NCLEX-PN CAT really is, how it is developed, how it is administered, what content is likely to be tested, and how it is scored. Graduate practical/vocational nurses must avoid the common pitfalls of failure, which include:

- A lack of understanding of what the NCLEX-PN CAT tests for
- An inability to realize how multiple choice questions are developed
- Not developing an effective study or review plan
- Underpreparing for the NCLEX-PN CAT
- Disbelieving they are smart enough to pass the NCLEX-PN CAT
- Overstudying information that is not likely to be tested on the NCLEX-PN CAT
- Not being able to control their anxiety before and during the NCLEX-PN CAT

The most effective way to become a better test taker and avoid the pitfalls described above is to *understand the rules of the game.* How many people play a card game, a computer game, or even a competitive sport without knowing the rules? Not many, yet a number of graduate nurses take the chance of sitting for the NCLEX-PN CAT (one of the most important tests of their life) knowing little, if anything, about how it works and what the rules are.

The NCLEX-PN CAT is an examination that all graduates must take and *pass* to practice as a licensed practical or vocational nurse (LPN/VN). The examination is a national examination developed by the National Council of State Boards of Nursing, Inc. (NCSBN) and is administered in testing centers throughout the United States. The NCSBN was founded in 1978 to develop licensure examinations for practical and vocational nurses and registered nurses that would reflect a minimal level of safe practice to guard consumers from incompetent graduates.

The NCSBN (which is comprised of representatives from all the state boards of nursing in the country, District of Columbia, and U.S. territories) develops the examination for licensure, while each individual state board and territory board is responsible for regulating, licensing, and disciplining nurses within their jurisdiction. The boards of nursing are responsible for regulating all nursing practice in their jurisdiction. This accounts for some of the differences in the exact role of the LPN/VN in various states and locations, because the scope of practice is defined by each state/territory board.

The NCLEX-PN CAT examination is designed to be based on job performance studies conducted by the NCSBN. The most recent study was completed in 1994 and describes the characteristics of the entry-level practical/vocational nurse, their practice activities (role activities), and their work environment.[1] In the study, 3,600 entry level LPN/VNs were surveyed about their practice activities. The framework for this study followed the previous one, which was performed in 1985. The study results then become the blueprint for determining areas of practice and activities that entry level nurses perform and which should be included in the NCLEX-PN CAT. To accomplish this, the results of these job performance studies are compared with the test plan to determine if the examination is actually testing "entry-level practice."

The test plan has been developed to reflect (1) the nursing process and (2) areas of client needs. An educational committee known as the "Examination Committee" decides the specific areas to be tested and the grading (weighting) assignment by category, which directs "item writers" (the nurses who write the examination questions) on where to generate questions in relation to the specific areas.

The NCLEX-PN CAT test is

◀ **What This Examination Is and What It Is Not**

- A measure of your understanding and application of the nursing process

- A way to determine your level of competence in nursing practice

- The method to protect health care consumers from unsafe graduates

The NCLEX-PN CAT test is not

- A way for you to better understand your strengths and weaknesses
- A test to teach you more about nursing practice
- An examination you want to take more than once

Let's take a closer look at the meaning of each of these statements to assist you in understanding this examination.

What it is:

■ **A measure of your understanding and application of the nursing process**

This means that you will be asked questions within a nursing process framework as defined by the NCSBN which may be slightly different than the way you have learned it (see section on Categories of Testing for the NCLEX-PN CAT).

■ **A way to determine your level of competence in nursing practice**

This means that your knowledge will be tested against other nurses who have successfully passed the NCLEX-PN CAT. It is also important to understand that this examination is a national examination that tests nursing practice competence throughout the country. This means that whatever nursing actions are being done in practice in White Fish, Montana must also be practiced the same way in Baton Rouge, Louisiana, San Diego, California, and Norwalk, Connecticut.

■ **The method to protect health care consumers from unsafe graduates**

The main justification for the existence of the NCSBN is to determine whether *you* possess the knowledge and judgment required in providing safe nursing care that will "do no harm," as Florence Nightingale said.

This examination is not designed for teaching or learning or to offer you insight into your nursing practice other than previously described.

What it is not:

■ **A way for you to better understand your strengths and weaknesses**

This examination is not designed to provide you with any information other than whether you passed (and can now be licensed) or you failed (and cannot now be licensed). It is not meant to be a learning-designed experience. Remember, the NCSBN has only one major reason to exist—to determine whether you have the competence to practice or not. The NCSBN provides candidates who did not pass with an individual diagnostic profile that allows them to see how they scored in the areas tested.

■ **A test to teach you more about nursing practice**

The NCSBN is attempting to determine "minimum (or safe) entry level nursing practice" for each candidate. They have established the passing score and are concerned only with whether the candidate's score exceeds this "minimum" or falls below it. They don't care if you score 100% or score one question above the passing standard. When you receive notification of passing the examination, if you passed by one question over the minimum passing score, it doesn't say "Candidate Passed—*barely*"; it simply says "Candidate Passed."

■ **An examination you want to take more than once**

The only thing you want to learn from this examination is that you never will have to take it again. This test will take all of your strength and concentration and requires a great deal of time to prepare for. Having to gear up a second, third, or even more times becomes more difficult with each attempt. So, let's try to get it right the first time!

SUCCESS RATE FOR THE NCLEX-PN CAT

The NCLEX-PN CAT was first administered on a national basis in April of 1994. Prior to computerization, the examination was administered two times per year and took a full day to complete. The advent of computerization allows the examination to be taken more than twice per year and is much more convenient than the previous paper and pencil test. The NCSBN reports results quarterly (four times per year) and annually with a summary of results. They report on several categories of testers, including first-time, U.S.-educated graduates; repeat, U.S.-educated graduates; first-time, foreign-educated graduates; and repeat, foreign-educated graduates. The pass rate for first-time, U.S.-educated graduate nurses in 1995 was 90.8%, and the pass rate for first-time, U.S.-educated graduate nurses in 1996 was 90.6%. Figure 1–1 demonstrates the number of first-time, U.S.-educated graduate nurses taking and passing the NCLEX-PN on the first attempt while Figure 1–2 shows the passing percentage for this same group.

The pass rate for first-time, foreign-educated nurses was dramatically different. In 1995, the passing percentage of first-time, foreign-educated testers was 54.1% and in 1996 the passing percentage was 54.7%. Fig-

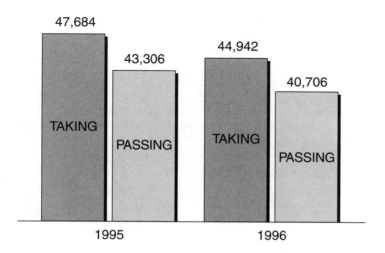

FIGURE 1–1. First-time, U.S.-educated graduating practical/vocational nurses taking and passing the NCLEX-PN CAT.

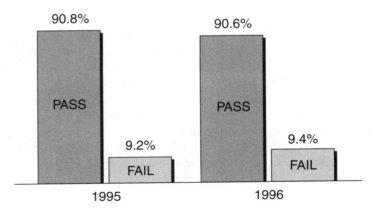

FIGURE 1–2. Passing rates: First-time, U.S.-educated graduating practical/vocational nurses.

ure 1–3 demonstrates the number of first-time, foreign-educated graduates taking the examination and the number passed. Repeat takers had an even lower success rate. In 1996, only 47% of the repeat, U.S.-educated testers passed (Figure 1–4), and only 25% of repeat, foreign-educated testers passed (Figure 1–5). (Source: Brown, V., Yocum, C., White, E. (1997). *1995–1996 Licensure Statistics.* Chicago: National Council of State Boards of Nursing, Inc.)

CATEGORIES OF TESTING FOR THE NCLEX-PN CAT

The NCLEX-PN CAT is structured to test two components of nursing practice: action and care. The action component is based on the phases of the nursing process, and the care component describes the client needs category. The weighting of the examination changed in October of 1996 and was based on the report and recommendations generated by the nursing job study mentioned previously. The *nursing process* category includes Data Collection, Planning, Implementation, and Evaluation. The *client needs* category includes safe, effective care environment; physiologic integrity; psychosocial integrity; and health promotion and maintenance. It is important to understand the weighting of each of these categories, because it will help you understand what is being tested and can help you approximate the areas that are tested more heavily than others.

Nursing Process Components ▶ **Data Collection**

This area is clearly described. It includes the assessment component of your nursing practice. Data collection involves three major areas: gathering information about the patient/client and significant others; being able to communicate the findings of data collection appropriately; and using the data collected to assist in the development of a therapeutic plan. Questions in this area are generated to focus on client interviews, family and significant other interviews, obtaining information from previous records and other health professionals; being able to distinguish which findings are normal and which are abnormal (and what the abnormality may mean), including the results of diagnostic tests; and collecting additional information to establish problems and potential problems. In other words, this section tests whether the nurse can obtain

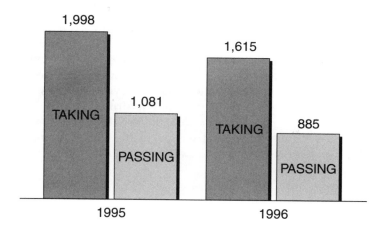

FIGURE 1–3. First-time, foreign-educated graduating practical/vocational nurses.

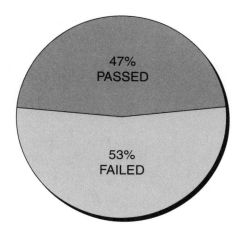

FIGURE 1–4. Repeat, U.S.-educated graduating practical/vocational nurses. January 1, 1996 through December 31, 1996.

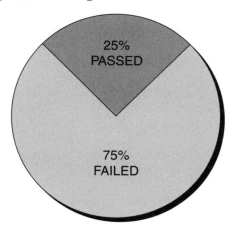

FIGURE 1–5. Repeat, foreign-educated graduating practical/vocational nurses. January 1, 1996 through December 31, 1996.

appropriate information in a given situation, recognize when something is not right, and know when there is a need to acquire additional information. Questions will also determine your ability to communicate normal from variations in normal in medical records or documents and to other health care providers. Finally, this section will test your ability to organize the data to assist in the care plan development by knowing the relationships between the significant information you have collected and the health problems (or potential problems) they may represent. This area carries substantial weight in the examination, because the number of questions will be between about $1/4$ (27%) and $1/3$ (33%) of your examination.

Planning

Planning includes two major areas: being able to assist in development of goals for the client/significant others to facilitate care, and to assist in the actual development of the nursing care plan. Activities associated with planning include determining and communicating ideas about nursing interventions that can be used to best meet individual goals; getting the clients and significant others involved in the development of the plan; adapting or individualizing nursing interventions to better meet client needs; devising a plan that will ensure the safety of the client/significant others and provide for the greatest comfort; and maximizing the potential of the individual or significant other. Questions in this area include establishing priorities of care within the plan, assisting in the formulation of the plan of care, determining the appropriate interventions in specific situations, planning ways to ensure a safe environment, and determining ways to maximize client potential. Another consideration includes the involvement of the client and significant others in care plan development. The weighting of this area is lower than the data collection area and will range from a little less than $1/5$ (17%) to $1/4$ (23%) of your examination.

Implementation

This area of the nursing process is defined by three major frameworks: assisting in nursing management of the client; providing care that will help to meet the established goals of the client/significant others; and communicating/documenting information pertinent to the care provided. Activities associated with implementation include implementing the care plan; participating in client care conferences; using a safe approach and established techniques in care delivery; getting the client ready for procedures; determining untoward reactions to interventions; acting appropriately in emergency situations; encouraging the client to participate in his or her care and to comply with the plan of care; monitoring client care provided by nursing assistants and other unlicensed health care providers; documenting interventions and the client responses and reactions to the interventions; and reporting pertinent information to other health care professionals. Questions in this area can include items related to implementation of care, documenting care and the client responses to it, noting and communicating any health status changes in the client, and recognizing and using the strengths of a client/significant other in meeting the nursing care plan goals. This area is heavily weighted the same as data collection (27 to 33%).

Evaluation

This portion of the nursing process expects that the nurse will be able to determine whether the client is able to meet the outcomes established in the plan. It will include suggestions for revision of care and the nurse's ability to report and document the client's response to interventions, treatments, and procedures. Evaluating compliance to the nursing recommendations and plan and understanding of client teaching is also part of this section. Questions in this area include determining if the client has met the goals established; reviewing the effectiveness of specific interventions; identifying areas of the plan that require revision; and recognizing the response of the client when performing therapeutic interventions. This area is weighted similarly to planning (17 to 23%).

Safe, Effective Care Environment

◄ **Client Need Components**

This category ranks number 2 (16 to 22%) in terms of information to be tested and includes the safe delivery of care and interventions; considering and maintaining an environment free of hazards; and coordinating care for clients/significant others. Questions included in this area focus on preserving the privacy and dignity of the client; supervising the delivery of care by nursing assistants; collaborating with health care team members and participating in nursing care conferences; and acting to prevent unsafe care delivery. In terms of a safe environment, the questions could include items testing the understanding of advanced care directives; the concept of informed consent; proper identification of clients; use of universal precautions; following infection control and biohazard policies; protecting the client from injury; and reporting environmental hazards, including faulty equipment. Other procedure-related topics tested include the proper methods for obtaining specimens; maintaining sterile technique; client education about treatments and procedures; determining the level of understanding of clients/significant others; and monitoring clients after procedures.

Physiologic Integrity

This area of client needs is weighted the heaviest of all. Almost 1/2 (49 to 55%) of your examination will be testing this category. Three major concepts make up this category: providing appropriate basic care; recognizing and decreasing the client's risk for developing complications from treatments, procedures, or medications; and providing and delivering care during emergencies, acute disorders, and chronic diseases. Questions in this area are directly related to understanding the principles of fundamental nursing care such as giving sitz baths; application of heat/ice per prescription; monitoring health status via vital signs; and providing for specific treatments such as tracheostomy care, suctioning, wound and decubitus care, medication administration, implementing comfort measures, and providing adequate nutrition. Examples of emergency care include CPR; administering oxygen; identifying alterations in health status (before, during, and after procedures and diagnostic tests); and assisting the client via Ambu bags. In the area of decreasing risks for clients and others, items could include proper range of motion; application of support hose; testing capillary blood glucose levels; measuring output of urine, stool, and drainage; administering and monitoring the effectiveness of medications including pain management; maintaining proper nutrition, fluid balance, and skin integrity; and assessing intravenous infusion sites. Cast care, nasogastric suction, and assessment of various systems (eg, cardiac, respiratory, GI) are also part of this area. Providing basic care includes bowel and bladder management, ostomy management, use of crutches, ambulation, and activities of daily living. Other areas include assisting with eating, obtaining accurate weights, and providing for rest.

Psychosocial Integrity

This area of client needs carries the least weight, and the examination will contain a little less than $1/7$ (8 to 14%) of the questions. This category addresses how the nurse incorporates principles of adaptation, coping, and mental health care during times of stress, illness, and loss. It also includes knowledge of common disease processes within the mental health spectrum, including chemical dependency. Spirituality and cultural beliefs are included in this area. Mental status assessment and therapeutic communication are also tested within this category. Examples of topics tested would likely include the ability to assess for reality and reality orientation; knowing signs and symptoms of withdrawal from chemicals; managing violent, aggressive, provocative behaviors; caring for the issues related to death and dying and grief and grieving; and identifying anxiety, body image disturbances, and coping patterns and methods used in stress reduction programs.

Health Promotion and Maintenance

Growth and development, the ability to care for self, support systems, disease prevention, and early intervention are the major concepts tested within this category (15 to 21% of the examination). The types of questions likely encountered would include items such as health screening programs; client education about early signs and symptoms of diseases; teaching positive health behaviors such as weight reduction and smoking cessation; interpreting skin tests; providing emotional support to families and clients experiencing chronic diseases; assessing client readiness to learn; assessing and providing care to the newborn; evaluating growth and development; and managing the mother in the labor and delivery process. This area would also include teaching prenatal care, parenting skills, and self-medication.

TAKING THE NCLEX-PN CAT EXAMINATION

The National Council of State Boards of Nursing, Inc. (NCSBN) has been given the responsibility to determine the competency of nursing program graduates who wish to practice nursing. Their duty is to

1. Determine what "entry-level practice" is

2. Develop a way to measure entry-level practice

3. Regulate the standards that are required for entry-level practice

The NCSBN does not issue licenses to practice. That responsibility is left to the states and territories in which the graduating nurse would like to practice. The individual state boards will issue a license when the candidate for licensure has demonstrated competence to practice.

This is evidenced by graduating from a nursing program that has been approved by the individual state boards in which the nursing program is being conducted and by demonstrating a successful passing score on the NCLEX-PN CAT examination.

The information on which you will be tested looks at your ability to provide what is described as safe, effective nursing practice (or a level of practice that demonstrates nursing knowledge related to established standards set by the NCSBN). Different cognitive levels of thinking are tested using the information you obtained in your nursing program. Three cognitive levels—knowledge, comprehension, and application—are tested.

This level of question is considered the easiest form of information to test for. It includes data which you have learned and probably memorized. The following example is a knowledge-based question.

◀ **Knowledge-level Questions or Items**

The normal heart rate of a 45-year-old adult would be considered to be within the range of
A. 30 to 59 beats per minute
B. 60 to 99 beats per minute
C. 100 to 139 beats per minute
D. 140 to 179 beats per minute

Knowledge-based questions are perhaps the easiest type of questions to answer because they are looking for your knowledge of a factual piece of information. I could teach my 14 year old the correct answer, and he doesn't have to even know what a pulse is. This realm of information is acquired by the learner from memorization. (By the way, the correct answer is B, because the parameters of a normal heart rate falls between these numbers. Answer A is known as bradycardia; answers C and D are described as tachycardia.)

This level of questioning is more complex. Rather than asking the candidate to know the facts, they may be asked to determine which is the most important fact or piece of information. For example:

◀ **Comprehension Level Questions or Items**

Which of the following would be considered a sign of right heart failure?
A. shortness of breath at rest
B. producing pinkish, frothy sputum
C. not being able to lie flat
D. edema of the feet and legs

If this question appears a little more difficult for you, don't get discouraged—it is. Look at the answers; each of these is a sign or symptom of heart failure. However, answers A, B, and C are symptoms (A) and signs (B and C) of left heart failure, while answer D is the only sign of *right* heart failure. This level of question asks the candidate which of all of the findings presented in the answers is associated in right heart failure first. If you were able to pick up the key word (*right*) and have the knowledge base to determine right from left heart failure signs and symptoms, then you would be able to answer this question correctly. You must recognize key words.

Application-level Questions or Items ▶ This type of question is the most complex level to be tested on the NCLEX-PN CAT. It requires you to take the information provided and decide which answer would be appropriate within that specific situation. For example:

> *Which of the following would the nurse do **first** for the client in bed who has a history of congestive heart failure and is experiencing sudden shortness of breath?*
>
> A. Call for more help.
> B. Assess the client's pulse rate.
> C. Sit the client up in the bed.
> D. Suction the client orally.

As you can see, all of these actions appear to be part of the nursing approach to be taken for management of the client who is experiencing shortness of breath, but in this specific situation, you should know to sit the client up to improve his or her airway and breathing (C). Answer A would be appropriate immediately after answer C (but you would not leave this client); answers B and D would be actions which might be taken soon after C and A, but would not be expected to be done *first.*

If you noticed that each of the last three questions became more thought provoking as you read them, it is because each question required more thinking and decision-making skills than the previous one.

REGISTERING AND TAKING THE NCLEX-PN CAT

Prior to April 1994, the NCLEX-PN was a full-day marathon which was completed in two sessions. It was administered by paper and pencil (fill in the little bubbles using a number 2 pencil) twice per year in April and October. The nursing program graduate could practice as a "graduate nurse" or GN until they sat for the first examination they were qualified to take, and until they received the results of this examination. In April 1994, the NCSBN changed the examination format to a computer "adaptive" examination, which means that the examination is now interactive and designed for each individual test taker. The test is administered by Educational Testing Service (ETS) and offered at Sylvan Testing Centers. There are over 150 test sites throughout the United States and territories that are open six days per week (and sometimes may be open seven days, depending on needs). Prior to applying for a testing time, you must establish your eligibility to sit for it. The process starts by applying to the board of registration in nursing for the state in which you wish to practice. The application must include evidence that you have graduated from an approved practical/vocational nursing program. Upon graduation, the nursing program will supply this evidence to you or the state board you select. The state board will review this information and make a decision to allow you to sit for the examination. Approval will be returned by mail as an "authorization to test" along with additional information (Candidate Bulletin) instructing you on how to establish a testing date. Now, here is the great part: You can schedule to take the examination at any test location listed in the bulletin. If, for instance, you decide you want to travel or plan a lengthy (well-deserved) vacation, you can take the examination in the area where you are staying and have the results sent to the state where you want to obtain your nursing license and practice. In addition, you can schedule a time that is convenient for you. If you are a morning person, afternoon person, or evening person, you have the flexibility to tap into the time when you are the sharpest!

You will be required to wait at least 30 days after graduation to take the examination and will be offered an appointment within another 30 days of your phone call. Hence, new graduates will be able to take the NCLEX-PN CAT within two months of graduation. Repeat testers will have to wait 90 days from their previous test and will be scheduled within 45 days from their phone call (providing it is longer than the 90-day requirement). Prior to 1994, you may have heard the term "graduate nurse" or GN which was given to those waiting to take the written examination. This GN status no longer exists because of the short time in which you can obtain a license via this process. It was also abolished because it would be impossible to track when each individual nursing graduate took his or her examination and either passed or failed. Some nursing graduates I have encountered have waited 3, 6, and even 12 months after they graduated to take their test (not a time period I would recommend for most candidates). As a result, if there continued to be a GN status, some people could practice nursing for long periods without ever taking the examination.

You will be required to pay all fees when you register for the NCLEX-PN CAT. Should you need to cancel or change the scheduled date, you can do so without penalty (or additional cost) up to three business days prior to the examination. Cancellation of your test date within three business days will result in your loss of the testing fee and require you to go through the scheduling process again. If you fail to show up for the examination, you forfeit all fees regardless of circumstances.

The test site will advise you to arrive at least 30 minutes before the scheduled time of the examination (this will reduce some of the anxiety as well). Arriving later than 30 minutes before your scheduled time may jeopardize your sitting for the examination and create registration problems (which can be very anxiety provoking). You should also keep your belongings to a minimum. You will be provided with a locker or a safe place to store anything you bring, but by keeping personal valuables to a minimum, you will not have the additional distraction of worrying what might become lost or stolen.

Here are several important reminders to keep in mind when coming to the test site.

1. Make sure you are there *on time*. (Don't set yourself up for failure before you begin.)
2. Make sure you bring *two forms of identification* with you. It is advisable (in fact, required) to make sure that each identification source has your signature and your picture on it. Items such as drivers' licenses, passports, employee identification badges, and school identification badges/cards are considered acceptable forms of identification by the NCSBN and testing center.
3. Make sure that your forms of identification have the *same name* you used to register for this examination. For example, if your driver's license says you are Jane Patricia Rogers, then register for the exami-

nation that way (if you plan to use your driver's license as your primary identification source). Also, whenever you correspond or contact the NCSBN or the Sylvan testing center, use your name exactly as it is written on your application.

4. *Do not change your name* at any time during this process!!!!!!! You will not be granted admission if your identification does not match your application name. If you are married, divorced, or adopted and change the identification you carry, it will not be accepted, and you will not be admitted to take the examination.

5. The testing center will *take a picture of you* when you are registering for the examination. This picture is entered into your registration record, and obtained for security purposes to assure that you are the person you say you are.

6. You will also be thumbprinted for identification purposes, and your thumbprint will be entered into your registration record for security purposes.

After you have completed the registration process, and at your scheduled time, you will be allowed to enter the testing area to your assigned test station (each testing site has at least 10 wheelchair-accessible stations). Each station is 30 inches deep by at least 48 inches wide. You will be provided scratch paper to make calculations which will be collected upon completion of the examination. You will not be allowed to take anything or anyone (other than yourself) into or out of the examination room.

The examination will take a maximum of 5 hours to complete. Included in the 5-hour period is a short tutorial designed to familiarize you with the NCLEX-PN CAT method of testing, a required 10-minute break after two hours of testing, and an optional break after another $1^1/2$ hours of testing. To leave the testing area you must sign out and sign in upon return. Two variables will decide how long your test will be. The first is the length of time you spend on each item/question; the second is the amount of items/questions you will be required to answer. You may be seated with a group taking the NCLEX-PN CAT at the same time, but each tester may finish the examination at a different time. Some testers may be finished after the minimum 85 questions; others may be required to answer the total 205 questions; and still others may be finished anywhere between the minimum (85) and maximum (205) number of questions.

Not all of the first 85 questions count toward your score. Some of the items in the first 85 questions are being tested for use on future examinations and are being tried out on you to see how good/effective/clear they are. This is how the NCSBN establishes reliability and validity for each question in the item pool from which the computer selects. Each item that counts on your examination has gone through the same process to establish a level of fairness.

One important point to remember is that this examination is interactive. It is designed for you as you answer questions. If you get the first answer correct, the computer will select one slightly more difficult. If you get the first answer wrong, the computer will select one slightly easier.

The third question is selected based on your second response the same way, and so on throughout the test. You must answer each question in the order it is presented so that the computer can offer you the next question. You cannot go back to previously answered questions. The computer is attempting to determine your level of competency based on the answers you provide. As you answer more difficult questions or easier questions, the computer will begin to establish a specific level of difficulty at which you are consistently scoring. As a consequence, it is a number of questions which will establish your fate, and no single question will have any greater weight in the examination than any other question.

The NCSBN draws an analogy between the NCLEX-PN CAT and a foul-shooting contest. The free-throw line represents the passing standard, and your test begins in front of the foul line (closer to the basket). If you answer the first item correctly, then you are moved slightly away from the basket and closer to the free-throw (or passing) line. If you answer the first item incorrectly, you are moved slightly closer to the basket and further away from the free-throw (passing) line. Your next shot will determine your next position. Make the shot and you will be given a slightly more difficult shot (question) to make; miss it and you will be given a slightly easier shot (question) to make. This continues until you are either making shots beyond the foul-shooting line (or correctly answering questions significantly above the passing standard) or until you are not making any shots near the free-throw line (answering questions incorrectly and significantly below the passing standard). No decision, either pass or fail, will be made until you have answered at least the minimum number of questions (85).

◀ **The Free-throw (Foul-shooting) Explanation**

In addition, there are several other ways to determine passing or failing this examination. For instance, you can still pass the examination if you answer the maximum number of questions and your competence level remains above the passing standard (even if it is not significantly above it) for the last 60 items you answered; or if you run out of time (and have answered at least the minimum number of questions) and the last 60 items answered were all above the passing standard. You will fail if you don't answer the minimum number of questions in the 5-hour period, or if you answered the maximum number of questions and you have fallen below the minimum competency level (passing line) at least once in the last 60 items.

With each response, the computer is making an analysis of your level. When the computer makes a statistically significant decision (in other words, when it can accurately predict whether you have passed or failed), the computer will end your examination (but you will not know whether you have passed or failed at that time). After the examination is completed you will be asked to complete a short questionnaire providing your input into the experience of taking the computer adaptive examination. Your examination results will be downloaded and sent to ETS by the end of that day, and they will process the information and notify your state board of nursing of the results within 48 hours. The state board will notify you of the results usually within 10 business days, but this varies from state to state (and time of year).

RUMORS, RANTINGS, AND RAVINGS

The closer you get to graduating and taking the NCLEX-PN CAT, the more myths and misconceptions you will hear. Some of these are out-and-out incorrect, and others are half-truths resulting from a misunderstanding of the process. The following are frequently passed rumors that you are likely to hear from a number of people.

Rumor Number 1: You know you pass when you answer the minimum number of questions and the computer shuts off.

This untruth is told repeatedly. In reality, you cannot make any prediction about whether you passed or failed based on the number of questions you have taken. It is true that more people who answer the minimum number of questions will pass than fail, but it cannot be predicted on an individual basis.

Rumor Number 2: You know you fail when you answer the maximum number of questions.

This is not true. It cannot be predicted whether you have passed or failed based on answering the maximum number of questions. (See the answer to the first rumor.)

Rumor Number 3: You know you answered a question wrong because the computer takes longer to provide you with the next question.

The computer may provide questions with various speed, but this speed is not related to whether your previous answer was correct or incorrect. It is more likely that any time delay in providing you with a question is based on the number of testers using the computer data bank or other variables not related to correct or incorrect answers.

Rumor Number 4: If you are not notified within 10 days, you probably failed.

This is not true! Most state boards have decided to notify candidates within 10 *business* days. Business days include Monday through Friday (excluding holidays), so you may not be notified for more than two weeks from the day you took your examination. You should check with your candidate bulletin and the individual state board to determine how long they routinely take to notify candidates of results.

Rumor Number 5: If you fail the examination, the next test will be much harder.

The computer knows whether you have taken the examination before by your identification number. It will then lock out all the questions you received in your previous efforts; consequently, you will always get different questions than the items you answered previously. The level of difficulty is no different whether you take the examination once or five times (although I don't recommend you try this).

Rumor Number 6: You can't change answers.

This area is frequently misunderstood. Although you cannot go back and change answers, you are allowed an opportunity to change an answer before it is locked in. The computer is activated by the enter key and the space bar. The space bar moves between the options (A, B, C, and D) and the answer is highlighted when you select one of these with the enter key. However, your answer is not entered into the computer until you press the enter key a second time. If you want to change your answer after you have highlighted it (by pressing the enter key once), you can change it by using the space bar to move to another answer, ending the highlighting of the previous answer.

MANAGE AND CONQUER YOUR TEST-TAKING ANXIETY

I have heard from many repeat test takers who felt so anxious before they took the NCLEX-PN CAT that they knew they had failed even before they finished the test. I once spoke to a graduate who said, "I knew I was going to fail the minute I saw the first question." Did anxiety play a role in this person's failure?

Most probably. Did this person know the level of anxiety he or she was experiencing? Probably not. Have you ever had to speak or present a report in front of your class or in a clinical experience? When you did this, did you find yourself talking while thinking to yourself, "My mouth is moving and words are coming out of it, but I'm not sure what I am saying?" Then you were experiencing what I refer to as the "out-of-body syndrome," because it seems as if someone else is doing the talking while you are standing there listening. Have you ever read a test item and realized that you didn't even comprehend what the question was asking about? This is another example of someone who is experiencing moderate to severe anxiety.

To conquer and control your anxiety and tap into that energy to your benefit, you must be able to recognize when you are experiencing anxiety and what level you are feeling. Answer the following question in a short sentence.

I get especially anxious when I _____

_____

_____

Now, make a list of the symptoms and signs of anxiety you experience in your life.

1. _____
2. _____
3. _____
4. _____

By writing down the situations that make you anxious and recording your symptoms and signs of anxiety, you are beginning to take control of anxiety by recognizing its causes and some of the triggers or warning signs your body provides that signal increasing levels of stress.

The stress and pressure we create on ourselves in the testing situation can have a negative effect unless we take control of it quickly. Anxiety has the potential to both help and hinder test-taking performance. Many test-taking experts agree that mild anxiety is good to experience when taking an examination. It sharpens our skills and thought processes and gives us a feeling of being ready to respond to the test. The signs and symptoms of mild anxiety include irritability and impatience, a sharpened visual sense (by dilating pupils), and a feeling of being focused. For example, have you ever been sitting in the classroom waiting for the test to be passed out and said to yourself, "I wish they would hurry up so we could get started!"? If you have said this, you are probably experiencing mild anxiety. As you feel a greater amount of stress, you may begin to experience a moderate level of anxiety. Moderate anxiety starts to alter your senses and can make you begin to experience a more narrowed perceptual field known as "tunnel vision" and mild gastrointestinal symptoms such as a feeling of "butterflies." This level of anxiety is not productive to test taking. Severe anxiety occurs when you are under high levels of stress and results in easily distractibility. The symptoms and signs of severe anxiety are those associated with panic, an urge to flee, a feeling of impending doom, and helplessness. They can also include severe tachycardia, shortness of breath, extreme diaphoresis, dry mouth, and gastrointestinal disturbances such as diarrhea.

**Decreasing Your Anxiety Level ▶
During an Examination**

There are many ways to reduce your anxiety level. Most of the techniques involve some form of relaxation response and visualization. The key to reducing anxiety during a test (once you recognize that your level is rising) is to employ a quick, effective method that does not take more than 15 to 20 seconds. *Remember, time is of the essence!* One method that has proven especially time efficient and effective for a number of graduate nurses I have taught is to visualize a stop sign. Here is how to do it, but remember if you are going to use it during a time of stress or anxiety, you should start practicing once or twice per day now. Close your eyes and picture the color of the stop sign, the octagonal shape, the white border surrounding the red sign, and the bold white letters. After you are able to see the stop sign in your mind's eye (your imagination), take a deep breath, moving your shoulders up to your ears to accent the air you are inhaling. After you have taken this deep inhalation, begin to slowly exhale while spelling the word S-T-O-P. Do this action three or four times and you will notice a decrease in the symptoms and an increased ability to concentrate. I am convinced that this is one of the most effective methods to decrease anxiety during an examination because the word has such a positive trigger mechanism for several reasons. First, when you were growing up, what were your parents always saying to you? Stop that! Stop that! Stop that! (auditory stimulus). Second, when you are traveling, how many stop signs do you see in a day (visual stimulus)? Finally, if you have ever worked on an Alzheimer's disease unit, you have probably seen stop signs on doors and exits. When a demented person (one who can no longer recognize him- or herself in a mirror or even read, for example) approaches a stop sign at an exit, he or she will look at it carefully and usually turn away from that door (long-term memory stimulus). So, begin to practice this at least twice per day for one to two minutes and the method will pay dividends when and if you need it during the NCLEX-PN CAT.

The only time someone told me it didn't work was during a presentation of this technique to a group of practical/vocational nursing graduates. After describing the process, we practiced it several times when one person in the back of the class raised his hand and said, "I'm sorry, but whenever I visualize a stop sign I get very aggravated." Needless to say, I was somewhat surprised and asked, "What is it about a stop sign that aggravates you so?" He replied, "I am a military police officer, and each time I close my eyes I see someone running through the stop sign." I paused at this point to regroup and think of another suggestion when suddenly a person sitting in the front of the room responded by recommending, "If he is a cop, then why don't you have him visualize a *Dunkin Donut* sign!" While creating humor in the group (including the military police officer himself), the recommendation seemed to satisfy him. So if the stop sign doesn't work for you (although it seems to work for a large number of people I have spoken to), then perhaps you should find "your own *Dunkin Donut* sign." Regardless of what you use as your focus, practice the method, practice the method, practice the method.

TEST FOR SUCCESS: PASSING THE EXAMINATION

◄ Start by Building Your Confidence

If you are going to be successful, you must think success! Have you ever wondered how some people accomplish so much more than you do? How many times have you asked someone, "Where do you find the time to do all those things?" These people actually have developed a style that frees them from thoughts of failure and helps them visualize themselves as being successful. As one philosopher put it, "Failure is not an option." In short, you must believe in yourself and the education you have been earning. You must begin to develop a mindset that pits us (you, your colleagues, your teachers, and me) against them (the "item writers," the statisticians, the psychometricians, and the members of the NCSBN). It is helpful to focus your effort on someone or something (in this case, the NCLEX-PN CAT). You now have a target and something tangible to shoot at and battle with. Believe me when I say, "This is not a friendly examination in which you are trying to learn anything but you passed."

Once you have focused your thoughts on success and conquering this examination, you should turn your thoughts to what your success will bring. Think about what you will be doing in six months. If you wish to work with old people, young children, childbearing families, or adults in general, see yourself doing it. Spend a few minutes a day fantasizing what it will be like to be a licensed practical/vocational nurse practicing in your area of interest. Visit the setting in which you wish to work to make your goal more concrete and real. Next, take an inventory of what you are good at. Do this by completing the following statement:

I am very good at _____

and

I know I can do _____

When graduating nurses start to study for the NCLEX-PN CAT, they may begin to panic, convinced that they know nothing. For these people, the glass is half empty, not half filled, and the fear of failure can become overwhelming. Think back on what you are good at, and remember your strengths, to maintain a better perspective.

From Now on, Think Like an Item Writer ▶

An item writer is the person trained by the NCSBN to write questions. Each question is referred to as an item (hence the term "item writer"). Item writers are recruited among faculty members (perhaps some of your teachers have written questions for the NCLEX-PN CAT) and nurses practicing in the field. The NCSBN has taken great pains to make people good at creating items and then puts them to work for a week. They are surrounded by books and must validate every answer (both correct and incorrect), using them as resources. It is an incredibly difficult process, and item writers are considered successful if they can create 25 good, usable items in one week. That is a rate of about one question for every 2 hours of thought and work. From now on, when your are practicing and preparing, look at an item (question), from a construction perspective just like an item writer would. Ask yourself three questions:

- *"Is the question written clearly?"* (Does it read clearly and unambiguously?)
- *"What type of question is it?"* (Is it a knowledge level, comprehension level, or application level?)
- *"Does the item writer know what he or she wants for the correct answer?"* (Don't make the mistake of saying, *"I* think the correct answer is . . ." Rather, start saying "I think the *item writer* would say the correct answer is . . .")

By asking yourself these questions every time you look at an item, you will come to think more and more like an item writer. Think like the person who wrote the item and you will have a better chance of answering it correctly!

Begin to Develop Your Clinical ▶ Reasoning Testing Skills

The thought of developing clinical reasoning testing skills may be somewhat intimidating, but all this means is that you need to think like the test writing experts! In other words, by working in this area, you can *begin to take control* of this exam rather than *letting it control you!!!!!* To think like an item writer, you must act like an item writer!

For instance, when you are presented with a multiple-choice question, first ask yourself, "Does this question test an issue of safe practice, physiologic integrity, psychosocial integrity, or health promotion and maintenance?" This is the first step in exerting your control over the question. Second, you need to imagine what issues the question could be testing you about. For example, read the following situation and list 4 points on which the item writer could test you.

> *Mr. Tulley has fallen down his icy porch steps. He is admitted to the orthopedic floor with a fractured left hip and placed in traction prior to surgery and casting.*

Now, write down four major ideas or concepts the item writer could ask you about regarding this client.

CONCEPTS THAT COULD BE TESTED:

1. _____

2. _____

3. _____

4. _____

Let us assume that I am the item writer of the above situation and compare my thoughts to yours. Think about the nursing process first. You should have asked yourself what data collection topics could be tested. Several important questions can be introduced to determine the test taker's understanding of CSMs (or checking for the circulation, sensation, and motion of the extremities), checking vital signs to assess for any potential bleeding, and assessment of pain. I could ask a question about planning care for this patient, including client teaching regarding cast care after discharge or working with Mr. Tulley's family about care after discharge. I might write a question about implementation which could include how to manage a client in traction or how the nurse could work to improve this client's intake to improve healing. I could ask a question in the area of evaluation by looking for the client's knowledge about the complications to look for after discharge (eg, infection, swelling, or pain). Finally, I could tie these questions into the categories of client needs such as safe, effective care environment by asking questions about proper alignment in traction, proper position of weights in traction, or how to assist the client to ambulate with crutches; or I may check the test taker's knowledge of the need to assess the client's mental status in the area of physiologic integrity.

How does your list compare with mine? If you picked up on any of the areas I did, then you have already begun to think like an item writer! Remember, great minds think alike!!!!!

I am always amazed at how little students and graduates know about the rules of multiple-choice questions and their mechanics. An understanding of them is an important step in gaining control of the examination itself, regardless of when you are taking it. Understanding the rules and mechanics can help you improve your score even when you do not know what the question is asking. People who gain this knowledge and understanding can utilize it along with specific test-taking strategies to become a "sophisticated tester." Some nurses understand how multiple-choice questions are structured and how they work on an intuitive basis. I never assume that any test taker has a strong intuition for this, however, and believe that most (if not all) test takers can learn and apply this information.

◀ **The Rules of the Game**

The first lesson to learn to improve your score on the NCLEX-PN CAT is to know the components of a multiple-choice examination question (or item): the situation, the stem of the question, the correct answer, and the distracter. The NCLEX-PN CAT contains no multiple multiple-choice questions. In other words, there will be only four answers to each question. You will not see answers like A. 1 & 2; B. 2 & 4; C. 1 & 3; and D. 1 & 4. Each question will be followed by only A, B, C, and D. Don't hope to find answers like "some of the above," "all of the above," or "none of the above," as they are not used in this examination.

◀ **The Multiple-choice Question**

The Situation

Some of the questions you have been exposed to in your nursing programs and may encounter on the NCLEX-PN CAT start with a short story, presentation, or scenario. These provide additional information about the client, the family, or problems being experienced, which may help guide the tester to better understand the question associated with it. In the NCLEX-PN CAT, the situations (when used) will be presented on the left side of the screen. These situations or client scenarios must be read and studied carefully. Each word in the scenario should be considered pertinent and relative because it is.

The Stem of the Question

The stem of the question is the focus of it. It may be preceded by a situation, in which case the stem will be presented in the upper right half of the screen; or it may be a stand-alone type that has no additional scenario. In the second case, it will occupy the complete top part of the screen. Stems usually come in two types. The first type is presented in the form of an incomplete statement and the second type a complete question. Look at the stem of the knowledge-level question we presented previously. This is the incomplete statement format. (For the options, refer back to the Taking the NCLEX-PN CAT Examination section.)

The normal heart rate of a 45-year-old adult would be considered to be within the range of

Now look at the next item stem and observe the differences (this question came from the same section).

Which of the following would be considered a sign of right heart failure?

This item has a question mark at the end and is a complete statement. In addition to understanding the two major types of questions, remember, you should not receive any "negative stem" questions. These types of questions (for example, questions that read "all of the following except") are discouraged, so you shouldn't encounter any of these question types. Finally, either type of question stem may be preceded by a situation.

The Correct Answer

The correct response is, in my opinion, the easiest part of this entire process to create. When an item writer creates a question, he or she usually has the correct answer (or concept) in mind. The NCSBN requires that all correct answers be validated by at least two sources. That means that before a question can ever get to you, it has been proven to be true by two or more nursing textbooks (which is why we validate the questions at the end of this book in a similar way as an item writer would).

Misconceptions About Correct Answers ▶

Misconception Number 1: Answer Length

Has anyone ever taught you to pick the *longest* answer or pick the *shortest* answer? Well, you can't pick the correct answer based on answer length on the NCLEX-PN CAT (item writers have heard the same thing). The answers, both correct and incorrect, will follow one of three patterns. The item answers will be either all short, for example,

A. chest pain
B. dsypnea
C. indigestion
D. dizziness

or they will be all long, for example,

A. recapping and disposing of all needles used properly
B. putting on gloves and gown when providing any care
C. wearing a shield-mask whenever in direct client contact
D. making sure all visitors put on gloves prior to entering

or there may be two short answers and two long answers, for example,

A. a radial pulse of 100
B. complaints of intense pain in the affected extremity
C. cool, pale fingers
D. tingling and numbness on the side of the injury

Misconception Number 2: Always pick answer C because it is correct more frequently

The answers to the items on the NCLEX-PN CAT are assigned randomly, so if you are making a completely blind guess, any letter has an equal chance of being correct. Only one type of answer is ordered in any specific fashion and it usually includes numbers (from least to most amount). For instance,

How many milliliters would the nurse draw from a 10-mL vial of Dilantin containing 1000 mg if the order called for a dosage of 300 mg of Dilantin?

A. .03 mL from the 10-mL vial
B. 3.0 mL from the 10-mL vial
C. 30 mL from the 10-mL vial
D. 300 mL from the 10-mL vial

The Distracters

Incorrect answers are known as distracters, because they are supposed to distract you away from the correct answer. A good distracter will trap a test taker who doesn't know the answer but will not distract the test taker possessing the knowledge to recognize the correct answer. Distracters must be plausible and realistic but not too tricky. Incorrect answers must be subtle, because a distracter that is unrealistic won't separate out those who don't know the answers from those who do know them.

How to Read a Multiple-choice Item

There are several ways to read an item. I recommend the following method. First read the situation, if one is presented. Taking your time, make sure you understand all of the terminology covered. Spend a few seconds visualizing the type of question you could be asked. Then, look at the question (if you anticipated it, you are already taking more control over it). Third, look at each and every answer, and determine whether any of them appeal to you immediately. Fourth, look at the question again and, if the answer you have selected still appeals to you, pick it. If not, then restudy each answer slowly and begin to employ some of the following strategies. Never make a blind guess on any question. You should have a reason for selecting each answer; otherwise, you are wasting or throwing away questions. *Remember, we do not want to give them any advantage over us!* You cannot skip any questions, so you must make your best choice for each item as it is presented. People possessing English as a second language may create the additional step of translating the situation, item, and answers into another language. The act of translation may change the meaning of words or expressions which can increase the difficulty of items, and must be done carefully and in a timely fashion. You should keep your time per question to less than 1 minute and 15 seconds.

STRATEGIES FOR TAKING THE NCLEX-PN CAT

The following list of strategies can be built into your test-taking approach if you use them during your study and practice them while taking tests. Most graduate nurses have never been taught these strategies because many faculty members are not aware of them all. I attended 10 years of college and never took a formal college-credit course on item writing. I venture to say this is probably true of most nursing teachers. To prove my point, how many times have you taken an examination and afterwards the instructor agrees to eliminate questions or accepts more than one answer to an item? This is because teachers who are not familiar with the rules of creating multiple-choice questions may have problems creating "good" distracters that do what they are intended to do. Additionally, it happens because your nursing instructors do not have the same luxury of testing their questions out on thousands of test takers like the NCSBN does.

The following strategies apply to many of the NCLEX-PN CAT questions in certain situations, because item writers may also use them to distinguish correct answers from distracters. Carefully read and reflect on each of these for a few minutes, and then begin to incorporate them into your study and practice.

STRATEGY 1: Read each client description (situation) carefully.

Have you ever looked at your examination in a review and said to yourself, "I knew that! Why did I pick that other answer?" The reason often lies in not reading the client description carefully. Remember one important fact: *Every word* written into a client description (the situation) is there for a specific reason. For example, as you read the situation, it might mention the age of the client. If it does, remember that they are not including it to waste space. Your response should be to immediately think about the developmental stage that person may be in (I prefer to use Erikson's 8 stages of development).

In addition, in the heat of battle, with added anxiety, it is possible to misread words. *Paralysis* can be misread as *plegia,* or *disoriented* could be misread as *disorder.* Take a look at these three triangles:

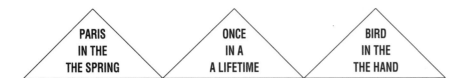

What does each of these expressions say? If you read "Paris in the spring," "Once in a lifetime," and "Bird in the hand," you have just made three "I knew that" errors. Look again. They read "Paris in the *the* spring," "Once in a *a* lifetime," and "Bird in the *the* hand." Reading too quickly, or not paying attention to every word will contribute to these types of errors. Don't fall into this trap; read every client description carefully!

STRATEGY 2: Do not "Yeah, but . . ." the question.

Remember the information provided is *the only information*. Many test takers read the question and begin to think too much about each answer. They start to think about what they have seen in their clinical experience, add extra information to the answer, or rationalize why a specific answer could be correct. Test takers who "yeah, but . . ." a question can talk themselves into almost any answer. Whenever you hear yourself looking at an answer and saying, "Yeah, but . . .," you are probably changing the intent of the question or answers. I love to talk to "yeah, but . . ." people in exam reviews because they usually say something like this: "Answer B is the correct answer." I reply, "No, the correct answer is A." The test taker then says, "Yeah, but if the patient were having difficulty breathing, then B is correct." (In the test situation, I never mentioned anything about the person having difficulty breathing; they added this information by reading too much into it.) I then say, "You're right. You answered *your* question correctly, but you still missed *mine*."

Let's look at a question the way someone would "yeah, but . . ." it.

When managing the client taking a fiber supplement such as psyillium, the nurse should

A. provide the medication immediately after breakfast
B. offer the medication when the client is going to bed
C. encourage the client to increase his or her fluid intake
D. assure the client that he or she will not have a daily bowel movement

Here is how I could "yeah, but" this question. Answer A could be correct because I have seen nurses in the nursing home giving it after breakfast; B could be correct because I have seen some clients who have taken this medication at bedtime; C could be correct because fluid intake is necessary when taking additional fiber; and D could be correct because most of the clients I have seen in the nursing home do not have daily bowel movements. Great!!!! I have just talked myself into every answer (by the way, the correct answer is C).

The major reason graduate nurses "Yeah, but . . ." questions is because they read too much into the item. If you have been working in a clinical role during your nursing education or have a great deal of health care experience, you are more likely to "yeah, but . . ." questions. If for example, you work with demented clients, then you might know too much about dementia and have seen too many variations or exceptions in your work. Remember, this is an entry-level practice examination, and everyone is being tested at the beginning level. When you go beyond this fact, you will tend to "yeah, but . . ." answers.

STRATEGY 3: Go with your first instinct; don't outguess yourself.

There will be many times (I hope) when you look at an item and are attracted to a specific answer. I recommend that you go with that answer, because first instinct responses are usually correct (provided you didn't make a misreading error). You will find that this type of feeling occurs in many items; when you feel it, go with the flow. Test takers will attempt to talk themselves out of first instinct answers by believing the answer is too easy. They say to themselves, "This answer is too easy. I must be missing something." You should trust your instincts and tell yourself that you are "on the same plane" as the item writer. Remember, great minds think alike, so don't talk yourself out of *first instinct* answers.

STRATEGY 4: Identify the nursing process category being tested.

The nursing process is a major concept being tested in the NCLEX-PN CAT. When test takers are able to determine what part of the nursing process the item is testing, they are at a distinct advantage. If, for instance, you can identify that the question is testing the "data collection" area of the nursing process, you can eliminate distracters that fall within other process categories. When practicing questions during your study, look for words that will identify the process area being tested. Item writers can easily mix "implementation" answers (distracters) in with "data collection" questions to determine if the test taker knows when more information should be collected before an intervention is performed. The following is a list of words that have been identified with each nursing process category. Look for them and use them to your advantage!!!

Data collection words:	observe	assess	identify	gather	recognize
	display	collect	detect	indicate	differentiate
	obtain	distinguish	describe	record	determine
	ask				
Planning words:	rearrange	formulate	plan	reconstruct	include
	generate	expected	criteria	short-term goals	prioritize
	outcomes	designate	categorize	set priorities	
Implementation words:	document	explain	give	inform	include
	teach	offer	administer	implement	encourage
	advise	provide	communicate	utilize	intervene
Evaluation words:	monitor	demonstrate	evaluate	synthesize	expand
	consider	question	determine	outcomes	conclude
	repeat	reestablish	compare	identify	

STRATEGY 5: Don't be distracted by previous questions; concentrate on the one you're looking at.

Each item requires your absolute concentration. One distraction having an adverse impact on your score is to remain fixed on previously answered questions. Test takers will continue to think about questions they answered five minutes ago and wish they could change the answers to those items. Well, you can't and if you focus on past items, you will get two questions wrong (the one you are looking at and the one you answered five minutes ago).

Another problem voiced by repeat takers is the distraction created when they receive a question that appears remarkably similar to one they just answered. The computer may select it simply because it is slightly easier or harder than the previous question without regard to the similarity of the item. Insecure test takers believe that they must have answered the previous question incorrectly, so the computer is asking it again to see if they will get it right this time. NOT SO. Any thoughts like this will serve to distract you from the question at hand. Remember, it is impossible to determine whether you answered the last question correctly or incorrectly. *Don't psyche yourself out! Stick to the current question!*

STRATEGY 6: Don't get angry because this will break your concentration.

Have you ever read a question during an examination and said, "This is stupid!" or "I wouldn't do any of these!"? If you have, then you have fallen into a major trap. By talking to the question, you are becoming inadvertently distracted and hence losing your concentration. Remember to *think* like an item writer. It is not what *you* think about the question or what *you* believe the answer to be. It is what you think the *item writer* thinks is the correct answer. Sometimes an item may touch upon controversial or potentially emotional topics such as rape, abuse, or the right to die. If you answer the question based on your own emotions or beliefs rather than what you think the *item writer* would believe to be the correct answer, you are making a huge mistake. Remember, this examination is not a test of your belief system or a format to make a social statement; it is a test of your nursing practice!

STRATEGY 7: Avoid choices with the words "always," "never," "all," or "none."

Extremes of words should put up a red flag. Very few situations in life are *always* or *never*, or *all* or *none*. These words give little leeway for any types of exceptions. Item writers may use these intentionally to make a distracter incorrect. In other words, a particular answer may be correct until the extreme word is added and makes it a wrong answer. Look at the following example:

Which of the following would be considered part of the management plan for the confused client who is wandering about the halls?

A. Ensure that the client is always being followed by someone.
B. Never let the client leave the care unit with his or her family.
C. Include only the client's family while teaching about wandering.
D. Observe and encourage the client to assist in his or her care.

Look at the words and tell me why A, B, and C are too extreme. You should notice the words *always, never,* and *only*. They are what make these answers less correct or incorrect. They represent the extreme.

STRATEGY 8: Look for answers that are somehow different.

Although item writers and the test development staff work hard to make every answer look the same, on a rare occasion they may overlook a difference. For example, if an answer contains a number (which makes it specific) and the other answers don't contain a number, look at it carefully because it is likely to be correct. Conversely, if one answer is not specific and the other answers are, look at it carefully, it is more likely to be correct. Here is an example:

> *When teaching a client about care of the skin during radiation therapy, the nurse would encourage the client to*
>
> A. cover the site with a dry dressing
> B. apply a thin layer of talcum powder
> C. use ice compresses to decrease pain
> D. wash the area with water once per day

Even if you knew nothing about radiation therapy, you may notice that answer D looks different. It has a frequency added to it (once per day) that the others do not have. Whenever you notice this, look carefully because it is often the correct answer.

STRATEGY 9: Look for priorities of care: Remember the ABCS.

When I see an indicator word such as "priority" or "do first," I immediately think about the ABCS (Airway, Breathing, Circulation, and Safety). Priorities of care are part of safe, effective practice and will analyze your ability to determine what should be done in the emergency situation. For example:

> *Which of the following interventions has the **highest priority** for the client experiencing a tonic–clonic seizure?*
>
> A. moving furniture away from the client during the seizure
> B. observing and recording the type and length of the seizure
> C. restraining the extremities to prevent injury or trauma
> D. turning the client on his or her side while loosening the collar

Always look for answers in this hierarchy. If there is an airway response in any answer, I usually pick it. If there is no airway answer, I look for and select the breathing answer. If there is no breathing answer, I look for and select the circulation answer. If there is no circulation answer, I look for a safety answer and pick it. The correct answer is D.

> *When managing a postoperative client who recently has undergone a radical neck dissection and tracheostomy for laryngeal cancer, which of the following would have the **highest priority**? The client is complaining of*
>
> A. loss of appetite with weight loss
> B. a change in the taste of foods

C. coughing and choking when swallowing
D. mild pain around the site of the tracheostomy

The correct answer is C. Answers A, B, and D are problems and complaints that need to be assessed. Coughing and choking when swallowing indicates the possibility of a tracheoesophageal fistula. An impairment of the airway needs immediate attention, as this can be a life-threatening situation as a result of possible aspiration. Now try this one.

Which of the following orders would the nurse question for the client who has just undergone a bronchoscopy?

A. Obtain vital signs hourly until stable.
B. Encourage PO fluids to 100 mL/h.
C. Make sure suction is available at the bedside.
D. Oxygen via nasal cannula at 2 L/min.

The correct answer is B, because the client should be NPO until the gag reflex returns. This answer is an airway answer and is one that the nurse would question.

STRATEGY 10: Look for answers that are client oriented.

What is your philosophy of nursing? Can you explain it in three words or less? Here it is. The secret to nursing is to *maximize client potential* (my opinion as it relates to the NCLEX-PN CAT). In other words, I am convinced that there is a hierarchy of responses to look for at all times. When these are included as part of the answer, I look closely at each.

LEVEL 1 RESPONSE

■ Look for answers that have the client doing something for him- or herself.

   (If there is no answer involving the client, move to the next level.)

LEVEL 2 RESPONSE

■ Look for answers that have the client's family or significant others doing something for the client.

   (If there is no answer involving the family or significant others, move to the next level.)

LEVEL 3 RESPONSE

■ Look for answers that have the nurse doing something for the client.

   (If there is no answer involving the nurse, move to the next level.)

LEVEL 4 RESPONSE

■ Look for answers that have another health professional (therapist, nursing assistant, physician) doing something for the client.

   (This is the lowest level of response and is used as a last resort.)

When reading questions, I look for answers that get clients to do something for themselves, or in other words, "Get clients involved with their own care and maximize their potential." (Level 1 response; if one is not there, look for level 2 responses, and so on.)

In addition, look for words that are facilitative. I've made a study of over 20,000 multiple-choice questions and have found the following words to be associated with correct answers:

assist	aid	support	encourage	facilitate
help	teach	foster	nurture	allow

Which of the following interventions would be appropriate for the client who is unable to produce any saliva?

A. Suggest that the person use a strong mouthwash prior to eating.
B. Recommend that the person add gravies and sauces with meals.
C. Encourage the person to drink several glasses of fluids with meals.
D. Tell the person that the use of hot foods will increase saliva production.

Isn't it much better to teach people than to tell them? Isn't it much better to encourage them than to suggest or recommend? Look for these words in answers and it will help you narrow your choices (especially if you have already narrowed it down to two answers). Answer C is correct because the nurse is *encouraging the person to do something.* Answer C is a double goody, because it uses a facilitative word (encourage) and gets the client to do something (drink several glasses of fluid with meals).

STRATEGY 11: Look for "indicator" words.

People often overlook indicator words. This type of words places a specific emphasis and dictates the urgency of the issue being tested. Here is a list of words to carefully look for in the question stem:

most correct	least correct	do first	do last
early sign/symptom	late sign/symptom	greatest priority	
least priority	most	least	

It is easy to miss indicator words during times of increased anxiety and make an "I knew that" type of error. Practice looking for these words in questions during your study and become more word sensitive.

STRATEGY 12: Try to turn answers into true–false possibilities.

This can be used as a final check before you hit the return key the second time. I will usually read the answer one last time and ask myself, "Is this statement true as it is written?" If I can assure myself that it is, I will stick to it; if not, I go back and look at the other responses again.

STRATEGY 13: Look for relationships between answers. Look for the broadest, most comprehensive answer.

Sometimes you may look at a question and say to yourself, "I like two answers and can't decide which I should select " (even after using all of the strategies in this section). In this case, look to see if one of the answers could be considered part of another answer. Look at this example.

Which of the following would be observed in the client who has been diagnosed with early cancer of the colon?

A. frequent, foul-smelling stools
B. clay-colored stools with blood
C. a change in normal bowel pattern
D. painful elimination with green-colored stools

You might have narrowed this question down to two answers (A and C). If you selected answer A, look again. Answer C says, "a change in normal bowel patterns." Answers A, B, and D are all changes in normal bowel patterns. Consequently, answer C is correct, because it includes all of the other answers. It is the broadest, most comprehensive answer.

STRATEGY 14: Select answers which are appropriate nursing actions.

Whenever you are presented with answers that are pharmacologically based or nursing intervention based, pick the nursing intervention. In other words, it is better to provide a therapeutic intervention (a sitz bath, for example), rather than acetaminophen for a person with hemorrhoids. (The only exception to this rule is when the person is in acute postoperative pain or is experiencing phantom limb pain.)

*Which of the following would be **most** appropriate for the postpartum patient experiencing perineal pain after delivery?*

A. administering aspirin 650 mg PO as ordered
B. assisting the client with a sitz bath
C. teaching the client how to do perineal exercises
D. reducing the amount and frequency of her stool softener

STRATEGY 15: Employ mnemonics to remember key points.

Use memory devices to remember specific facts or key points. For instance, remember the word **SWISS** as complications associated with persons who have Cushing's syndrome. It stands for **S**odium retention, **W**ater retention, **I**nfection potential, **S**ugar excess, and **S**econdary sex characteristic changes. Another example is: No **P** means no **K** (in other words, if the client is not putting out urine, do not give any extra potassium). Create your own memory devices as you study and send them to me so I can offer them to other graduates. (See the front section on how to contribute to this book.)

STRATEGY 16: Reschedule your examination if the test center experiences delays of longer than one hour.

On rare occasions, testers may experience delays in the administration of the examination. They may be scheduled for 9:00 A.M. but are not able to sit for the test until 10:00 A.M. for various reasons. Any delay longer than one hour is too long to wait. You should be at a mental peak when you begin taking this examination, and delays will increase your anxiety level and your fatigue level. Ask to have the examination rescheduled. The staff at the testing center are usually extremely accommodating in these regards, so you should have no difficulty having it changed without charge. Remember, don't accept any delays longer than one hour.

STRATEGY 17: Don't be distracted if you go beyond 85 items.

Many graduate nurses taking the NCLEX-PN CAT are convinced that if they go beyond the minimum number of questions, then they have failed. This is NOT true. All it means is that the computer has not yet arrived at a decision. If you begin thinking that you did not pass, because others are leaving while you are still answering questions, you will begin to lose control of the examination. Keep your cool and continue to answer the questions with the same intensity with which you started. More people who take the maximum number of questions pass the examination than fail, but only if they keep their heads and maintain control over it.

Develop a Pattern for Analyzing ▶ Questions and Answers

Now that you have been exposed to all of these strategies and information, how can you incorporate it into your test-taking bag of tricks? I recommend the following format:

1. Before you look at a situation, put your "item writer" hat on.
2. Clear your mind of any thoughts other than the test.
3. Read the situation first (if there is one) *carefully* and think about what you may be tested on.
4. Look for an age in the description.
5. Now look at the question. Recheck it for "indicator words."

   If they are present, begin to think ABCS if it is applicable.
6. Now read the answers, and if you have a first instinct, go with it.
7. If you can't make a choice or narrow it down to two answers, use this order to search for the answer. Look for
   - The nursing process being tested
   - Facilitative words
   - Words that are client/family oriented (think: philosophy of nursing)
   - The broadest and most comprehensive response
   - Answers which seem different
   - Words that are too extreme
   - "Nurse-appropriate" interventions

This is the pattern I use to answer questions, control the examination (rather than letting it control me), and narrow down possibilities even when I have no idea what the question is asking me. You can use this approach, adapt it, and even change it if you wish. What is important to remember is that whatever approach you use, make it a consistent one.

WHAT TO EXPECT AFTER TAKING THE EXAM

Once you have completed the examination, you will have to wait about 2 weeks for the results. The results will be sent by mail. The results are presented in one of two ways. If you passed the examination, you will receive an $8^{1}/_{2}$ x 11 page with your picture on it (the one they took at the exam site); some individual and program information such as your candidate number, date of birth, Social Security number, the nursing program code and name which you attended; and a statement which reads to the effect that you have passed the license examination. This statement is written in an area where the word NCLEX is presented in the background (Figure 1–6). If you don't pass the examination, you will get an 8¹/₂ x 11 sheet of paper with the same information at the top, but it will say that you have not passed, along with additional descriptions of the examination results. A diagnostic information section appears at the bottom half of the page which provides you with some data to see how you scored in the nursing process category and the category of client needs (Figure 1–7). On the reverse side of this page, you will find complete definitions of the nursing process and categories of client needs (Figure 1–8). You will also be supplied with additional information on how to register to retake the NCLEX-PN CAT.

REFERENCE

1. Chornick N, Yocum C, Jacobson J (1995). *Job Analysis Newly Licensed Practical/Vocational Nurses 1994.* National Council of State Boards of Nursing, Inc., Chicago, IL, 1995.

FIGURE 1–6.

NCLEX-PN™ CANDIDATE REPORT
National Council Licensure Examination for Practical Nurses

NATIONAL COUNCIL® — National Council of State Boards of Nursing, Inc.

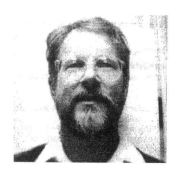

Test Date: MM/DD/YY
Test Center: X9999

Candidate Number: 123-12-678
Date of Birth: 12/31/58
Social Security Number: 123-45-6789
Program Code: 99-999
Program Name: SMALLTOWN COLLEGE OF NURSING
B   SMALLTOWN, OH

    WALTER P SMITH
    1234 MAPLE AVE.
    SMALLTOWN, OH 12345

WALTER P SMITH, an applicant for licensure by the MASSACHUSETTS BOARD OF REGISTRATION OF NURSING, HAS PASSED the National Council Licensure Examination for Practical Nurses.

FIGURE 1–7.

NCLEX-PN™ CANDIDATE REPORT
National Council Licensure Examination for Practical Nurses

NATIONAL COUNCIL® — National Council of State Boards of Nursing, Inc.

Test Date: MM/DD/YY
Test Center: X9999

Candidate Number: 123-12-678
Date of Birth: 12/31/58
Social Security Number: 123-45-6789
Program Code: 99-999
Program Name: SMALLTOWN COLLEGE OF NURSING
B   SMALLTOWN, OH

WALTER P SMITH
1234 MAPLE AVE.
SMALLTOWN, OH 12345

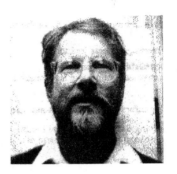

WALTER P SMITH, an applicant for licensure by the MASSACHUSETTS BOARD OF REGISTRATION OF NURSING, HAS FAILED the National Council Licensure Examination for Practical Nurses.

The scale below, titled "Overall Performance Assessment," shows how well you did on the NCLEX-PN. The "X" shows how far below passing your performance fell. Passing is indicated by the "|" shown in the box.

On the NCLEX-PN, no candidate is administered more than 205 questions. The box titled "Number of Items Taken" shows that the computer reached a decision after you had answered 205 questions.

"Only candidates whose performance was close to the passing standard, either just above or just below it, had to answer the maximum number of 205 questions. For candidates whose performance was much higher or much lower than the passing standard, fewer questions were required before a confident pass or fail decision could be made."

The back of this form lists the eight test plan content areas. The "X" in the eight boxes at the bottom of this page show how well you did in those content areas. This will help you know which areas to study before you take the test again.

OVERALL PERFORMANCE ASSESSMENT

	X	

<-------------------------------->
FAILING RANGE   PASS

NUMBER OF ITEMS TAKEN

							X

< 65   85   105   125   145   165   185   205

PHASES OF THE NURSING PROCESS
Data Collection (27-33% of the test)

X

<— lower performance   higher performance —>

Planning (17-23% of the test)

X

<— lower performance   higher performance —>

Implementation (27-33% of the test)

X

<— lower performance   higher performance —>

Evaluation (17-23% of the test)

X

<— lower performance   higher performance —>

CATEGORIES OF CLIENT NEEDS
Safe, Effective Care Environment (16-22% of the test)

X

<— lower performance   higher performance —>

Physiological Integrity (49-55% of the test)

X

<— lower performance   higher performance —>

Psychosocial Integrity (8-14% of the test)

X

<— lower performance   higher performance —>

Health Promotion/Maintenance (15-21% of the test)

X

<— lower performance   higher performance —>

415.07-09250/NRSPND-9/19/95

36

FIGURE 1–8.

NCLEX-PN® Examination Definitions

PHASES OF THE NURSING PROCESS
The four phases of the nursing process include:

I. Data Collection: Participate in establishing a database. (27% to 33% of the NCLEX-PN® examination)
   A. Gather information relative to the client.
   B. Communicate information gained in data collection.
   C. Contribute to the formulation of nursing diagnoses.

II. Planning: Participate in setting goals for meeting client's needs and designing strategies to achieve these goals. (17% to 23% of the NCLEX-PN® examination)
   A. Assist in the formulation of goals of care.
   B. Assist in the development of a plan of care.

III. Implementation: Initiate and complete actions necessary to accomplish the defined goals. (27% to 33% of the NCLEX-PN® examination)
   A. Assist with organizing and managing the client's care.
   B. Provide care to achieve established goals of care.
   C. Communicate nursing interventions.

IV. Evaluation: Participate in determining the extent to which goals have been achieved and interventions have been successful. (17% to 23% of the NCLEX-PN® examination)
   A. Compare actual outcomes with expected outcomes of client care.
   B. Communicate findings.

CLIENT NEEDS
The four categories of client needs are described as follows:

A. Safe, Effective Care Environment (16% to 22% of the NCLEX-PN® examination)

This category includes the client needs listed below:
   • Coordinated care.
   • Environmental safety.
   • Safe and effective treatments and procedures.

Knowledge, Skills and Abilities

Advance directives; communication skills; confidentiality; continuity of care; environmental and personal safety; expected outcomes of various treatments; general and specific protective interventions; informed consent; knowledge and use of equipment used to provide nursing care; legal accountability; quality assurance; client rights; spread and control of infectious agents; team participation.

B. Physiological Integrity (49% to 55% of the NCLEX-PN® examination)

This category includes the client needs listed below:
   • Physiological adaptation.
   • Reduction of risk potential.
   • Provision of basic care.

Knowledge, Skills and Abilities

Activities of daily living; basic pathophysiology; body mechanics; comfort interventions; effects of immobility; emergency interventions; expected response to therapies; fluid balance; invasive procedures; medication administration; normal body structure and function; nutritional therapies; pharmacological actions; skin and wound care; use of special equipment.

C. Psychosocial Integrity (8% to 14% of the NCLEX-PN® examination)

This category includes the client needs listed below:
   • Psychosocial adaptation.
   • Coping and/or adaptation.

Knowledge, Skills and Abilities

Behavior norms; chemical dependency; common treatment modalities; cultural, religious and spiritual influences on health; mental health concepts; therapeutic communication.

D. Health Promotion and Maintenance (15% to 21% of the NCLEX-PN® examination)

This category includes the client needs listed below:
   • Growth and development through the life span.
   • Self-care and support systems.
   • Prevention and early treatment of disease.

Knowledge, Skills and Abilities

Community resources; concepts of wellness; death and dying; disease prevention; growth and development through the life span; human sexuality; parenting; principles of immunity; reproductive cycle; teaching appropriate to the scope of practice.

Reprinted with permission of the National Council of State Boards of Nursing, Inc.

PART II

▶ High Index of Probability Items

- Cardiovascular System
- Respiratory System
- Hematologic System
- Endocrine System
- Gastrointestinal System
- Genitourinary System
- Special Senses
- Neurologic System
- Musculoskeletal System
- Immunologic System
- Integumentary System

Parts two, three, and four in *First Step for NCLEX Success* contain information which has been gathered from a variety of sources including faculty members, graduate nurses, student nurses, the NCLEX-PN job analysis study of 1994, and a variety of textbooks. The material presented in these sections should be considered essential information for anyone taking the NCLEX-PN CAT or preparing for other nursing examinations. These sections provide pertinent information, special ways to remember key facts and ideas, mnemonics, Safety Points, and additional selected facts covered in Points to Ponder to assist you in remembering essential points.

The information provided in each section is not meant to be comprehensive; rather it is meant to highlight important (high index of probability or "HIP" items) from procedures, diseases, disorders, treatments, diagnostic tests, psychosocial issues, pharmacology, maternal-child health care, care of children, and growth and development implications. Many graduate nurses need direction in separating out the *"need to know information"* from the *"nice to know information"* and the second, third, and fourth parts of *First Step for NCLEX Success* attempt to do this for you. Part 2 presents information in a body systems format including important A & P facts, assessment information, diagnostic tests, and procedures and nursing management information. Part 3 covers several specialties including maternal-child health, care of children, older adults, and psychosocial issues. Part 4 reviews pharmacological considerations by providing a group of medications and categories of medications which you are likely to encounter on the NCLEX-PN CAT.

If at times, the information provided to you in a given area may seem incomplete, it is because you are reading what we consider to be the most critical information needed to know in that area. If you have specific questions about a treatment (for example), you should go back to a nursing fundamentals book or a foundations of nursing text to reinforce the complete series of steps and rationales for performing the procedure or treatment.

We actively encourage graduate nurses, nursing students, faculty members, and staff to submit ideas, high index of probability items, and mnemonics as frequently as possible to expand and update these three parts. To do so, see the page on "How to Contribute."

Disclaimer

The information provided in these sections are the author's, graduate nurses', and nursing students' ideas and impressions of high probability items. We do not encourage, and strongly discourage, the submission of content or questions based on your personal experience with the NCLEX-PN CAT. All mnemonics are considered within the public domain, unless otherwise credited, and information printed in this section has been verified for accuracy using the traditional textbooks. Material submitted will be verified, if possible, with one or several sources. All errors and omissions will be gladly corrected if brought to the attention of the author through the publisher.

Heart Valves

- Four heart valves include the left-sided valves, the aortic and pulmonic, and the right-sided valves, the mitral and tricuspid.
- Damage to heart valves creates heart murmurs.

Pulses

Apical pulse

- Point of maximal impulse in heart.
- Used for obtaining the heart rate of clients taking cardiac medications or with irregular peripheral pulses.

Peripheral Pulses

- Upper: Carotid, radial, and brachial
- Lower: Femoral, popliteal, and tibial

Heart Rate and Rhythm

- Normal sinus rhythm is between 60 to 100 beats per minute and is a regular rhythm.
- Sinus bradycardia is less than 60 beats per minute and may indicate too much digoxin (digoxin toxicity), heart block, neurologic disorders, drug overdose, and hypothyroidism.
- Sinus tachycardia is greater than 100 beats per minute; can be caused by anxiety, adverse reactions to medications after a myocardial infarction, use of stimulants such as caffeine or cocaine overdose, hyperthyroidism, and with exercise.

Pallor

- When client shows a generalized pallor it could indicate conditions such as shock, blood loss, anxiety, myocardial infarction, infection, or other acute disorders.
- When the pallor is localized to the extremities only, it is usually a sign of peripheral vascular disease such as arterial insufficiency or arterial occlusion.
- Additional findings can include absent or diminished peripheral pulses, pain, and coolness or cold feeling when palpating the affected extremity.

Cyanosis

- A generalized cyanosis demonstrates poor perfusion or circulation from conditions involving the heart, blood vessels, lungs, or blood (anemia).
- When cyanosis is observed in the extremities only, it usually indicates peripheral vascular disease (arterial or venous insufficiency). Other findings may include edema, brown skin pigment, skin ulcers, or thickening of skin.

Edema

- Systemic or generalized edema is typically seen in disorders like heart failure, liver disease, renal failure, and hypothyroidism. Causes of localized edema include inflammation (cellulitis), obstruction of the lymphatic drainage system, and trauma in the involved area.

Data Collection, Procedures, ▶ and Treatments

Blood Tests

Serum Potassium

- Normal: 3.5 to 5.0 mEq/L.

CLINICAL NURSING IMPLICATIONS

- Increased levels occur with renal failure, high K^+ IV infusion, burns, and in metabolic acidosis.
- Low levels occur with diuretics, metabolic alkalosis, vomiting, and steroid use.

Serum Sodium

- Normal: 135 to 145 mEq/L.

CLINICAL NURSING IMPLICATIONS

- Increased in dehydration, renal disease, and too high a sodium intake.
- Decreased in vomiting, diarrhea, gastric suction, too much water intake, renal dysfunction, and overuse of diuretics.

Serum Digoxin Level

- Normal: 0.5 to 2 ng/mL for therapeutic effect.

CLINICAL NURSING IMPLICATIONS

- Note signs and symptoms of toxicity including nausea, vomiting, visual disturbance, yellow vision, and bradycardia.

Electrocardiogram (ECG)

- Records the electrical impulses in the heart and can detect cardiac irregularities and heart damage. Placement of electrodes will be on the extremities and in the chest area at the 3rd intercostal space on the right side, and the 3rd, 4th, and 5th intercostal spaces on the left side.

Stress Test

- This test measures symptoms and changes occurring with cardiovascular disease such as angina and myocardial infarction. Client walks on treadmill or rides bike.

▶ SAFETY TIP

Discontinue test if complaints of chest pain, lightheadedness, or vertigo are voiced. Also discontinue if cardiac irregularities develop. Have code equipment ready in testing area.

POINT TO PONDER

Never give potassium to any patient who is not voiding. No "P" means no "K."

POINT TO PONDER

Patients with low levels of sodium will present with acute onset of confusion.

Holter Monitor

- Used to measure heart rates and rhythms over a prolonged period of time, usually 24 hours, to rule out intermittent heart blocks or irregularities.
- No specific client teaching needed.

Cardiac Catheterization

- Used to evaluate the blood flow through the heart and the blood vessels of the heart

Preprocedurally

- Teach clients about the need to cooperate as they may be asked to cough during procedure.
- Clients may note a salty or metallic taste, palpitations, nausea, and a warm feeling when dye is injected.
- Procedure lasts one to three hours.

▶ SAFETY TIP

Chest pain when dye is injected is abnormal and should be reported immediately.

▶ SAFETY TIP

No aspirin or aspirin-like products for 7 days prior to procedure.

Postprocedurally

- Monitor vital signs every 15 minutes for one hour then every 30 minutes for two hours and then every hour for four hours.
- Pressure dressing and sandbag usually applied in procedure room to prevent hemorrhage.
- Check site for bleeding.
- Strict bed rest for 8 hours postprocedurally with head of bed elevated no more than 30 degrees.
- Strict bedrest for 6 to 8 hours.

Coronary Angioplasty (Percutaneous Transluminal Coronary Angioplasty)

- Performed in similar fashion as cardiac catheterization or in conjunction with a cardiac catheterization.
- Balloon inflated at end of cardiac catheter to open narrowed opening in a coronary artery.
- Discharge in 2 days.

POINT TO PONDER

Mark peripheral pulses for baseline.

POINT TO PONDER

Observe for bleeding or occlusion beyond the vessel used by checking peripheral pulses (especially the extremity that was used for the catheter) in the leg. If absent, notify physician immediately.

Central Venous Pressure (CVP) Monitioring

- Performed by placing end of cardiac catheter into heart to measure the pressure levels on the left and right side of heart.
- Decreased pressure indicates shock, and increased pressure indicates heart failure.

Cardiac Disorders ▶

Angina

- A condition that occurs when the heart does not receive enough oxygen. This typically occurs when the person is under increased stress or performing physical activity.

Data Collection

- Client may complain of pain on activity (relieved by resting), which is described as heavy, crushing, or dull; occurring over the sternum, epigastric area, jaw, back, and shoulders, and lasting for 1 to 5 minutes.
- ECG may change during episodes of chest pain.

Management

- Client teaching includes encouraging rest periods when chest pain occurs.
- Nitroglycerin (or other vasodilator) used to increase oxygen perfusion, and client teaching includes knowing whether the medication is effective. Client may note a headache, burning under tongue, and flushed feeling after taking medication.
- Nitroglycerin is stored in a dark, dry place for no more than 6 months.
- Instruct client to call ambulance if pain is unrelieved after three doses.

Myocardial Infarction

- This occurs when a blood vessel becomes totally occluded and results in tissue death beyond the obstruction.

Data Collection

- The pain may be similar to the pain of angina but usually doesn't have a relation to activity, lasts longer than 15 minutes, and may also include nausea, vomiting, diaphoresis, and pallor.
- ECG will usually be abnormal and cardiac enzymes will change after damage.

▶ SAFETY TIP

Advise client to call ambulance and not to drive to the hospital or have others drive them.

Management

- Administering oxygen per order will improve cardiac status.
- Medication given for pain (per order) is usually morphine sulfate. Thrombolytics (clot busters) are used to dissolve clots.
- Observe for signs of bleeding and check vital signs and stools for occult blood.
- Activities contraindicated after myocardial infarction include hot showers or baths or tubs, running in cold or hot weather, and heavy meals and excessive alcohol intake.
- Diet modifications include low-fat diet, with sodium restriction of 2 grams (no added salt).

▶ SAFETY TIP

Client teaching includes abstinence from sex for 6 weeks or until client is able to climb two flights of stairs without chest pain, tightness, or shortness of breath.

Comparison of Chest Pain in Angina and Myocardial Infarction

	Angina	**Myocardial Infarction**
Created and relieved by	Pain brought on by activity and relieved by rest and medication	No relation to activity and no relief from medications
Description	Heavy, crushing, dull	Heavy, crushing, dull
Location and radiation	Over sternum, epigastric area, jaw, back, and shoulders	Over sternum, epigastric area, jaw, back, and shoulders
Severity	Mild to severe	Mild to severe, but often includes a feeling of impending doom, nausea and vomiting, diaphoresis, and pallor
Duration of pain	Usually activity or stress related and lasts between 1 and 5 minutes	Lasts longer than 15 minutes with no specific activity relationship

Congestive Heart Failure

Data Collection

- Left-sided heart failure starts with complaints such as shortness of breath, orthopnea, and confusion.
- Right-sided heart failure starts with complaints of edema of extremities, or, if on bedrest, look for edema in coccyx area, distended neck veins, and fluid in the abdomen.
- Numerous crackles (rales) and wheezes can be heard throughout the lungs.
- Decreased urinary output/oliguria resulting in fluid retention.

> Weigh client daily, noting weight gain of more than one pound in 24 hours as significant (or more than 2 pounds in one week) one liter of fluid = 2.2 pounds of body weight = 1 kg of body weight.

Management

- Administer diuretics (as ordered) (usually Lasix/furosemide) and digoxin (as ordered); restrict fluids; administer oxygen (per order) and maintain a low-sodium diet.

Pulmonary Edema

- This is the most severe form of CHF and constitutes a medical emergency.
- When discovered, immediately sit the client up, stay with client, and call for help.
- Medical management may also include oxygen, morphine sulfate for pain and anxiety, diuretics, bronchodilators, applying rotating tourniquets, and monitoring blood pressure every 15 minutes until stable.
- Remember the words **MOST DAMP:**

    M = **Morphine sulfate**

    O = **Oxygen via mask**

    S = **Sit client up**

    T = **Tourniquets (rotating)***

    D = **Diuretics**

    A = **Aminophylline**

    M = **Monitor**

    P = **Pressure**

    *Rotating tourniquets: Rotate clockwise; change every 15 minutes. Pressure of tourniquet should be above diastolic pressure but below systolic pressure. When discontinuing, take one off at a time in 15-minute intervals (decreases potential for reestablishing CHF/pulmonary edema).

Shock and CPR

- Shock is a condition which results from failure of the heart, loss of blood, infections of the bloodstream, anaphylactic reactions, and spinal cord transection injuries.

Data Collection

- Early signs and symptoms include restlessness; anxiety; tachycardia; a drop in blood pressure; and cold, clammy skin.
- Late signs and symtoms include hypotension with low systolic pressure, a weak (thready) pulse, unconsciousness, tachycardia, and oliguria or anuria.

Management

- If cardiac arrest occurs, begin CPR:

    One-rescuer ratio: 15 compressions to 2 breaths

    Two-rescuer ratio: 5 compressions to 1 breath

- Check for unresponsiveness.
- Call for help.

- Establish airway (don't hyperextend neck; extend neck)
- Check for breathing for 5 to 10 seconds.
- Give two breaths if not breathing.
- Check for pulse for 5 to 10 seconds.
- Proper hand placement is 2 fingers above xiphoid in adults.
- Compressions are $1^1/_2$ to 2 inches in adults.

▶ SAFETY TIP

Stay away from bed and client when defibrillation is performed.

Valvular Disease

- *Mitral valve* disease is usually seen in women, with rheumatic fever being the most frequent cause. Signs and symptoms may include fatigue, dyspnea, and congestive heart failure (in severe disease).
- *Aortic valve* disease is usually seen in men, with rheumatic fever frequently the cause. Signs and symptoms can include angina, dsypnea, and exertional syncope (fainting).
- *Tricuspid and pulmonic valve* problems are much rarer but compare similarly to problems presented with the mitral and aortic valve, respectively.

Pacemakers

- Teach clients how to count their own pulse.
- Instruct clients to have pacemaker checked regularly by physician.
- Instruct clients to stay away from electrical fields such as microwave ovens, airport metal detectors, and high-tension wires.
- Instruct clients to carry a medical identification card and bracelet at all times.

Common Intravenous Infusion Complications

◀ **Vascular Disorders**

Complication	Signs and Symptoms	Nursing Management
Infiltration	Pain, swelling, and coolness at the site and around it	Discontinue infusion; elevate the extremity
Phlebitis	Pain, tenderness, and redness at the site, and along the blood vessel being used	Discontinue infusion; apply warm compresses to area
Thrombus	Delivery of fluid stops; pain, tenderness, and redness may occur at the site	Discontinue infusion; apply warm compresses to area; avoid palpating or applying pressure to area
Infection	Fever, inflammation, pain and tenderness, and drainage at the site	Discontinue infusion; change tubing every 24 hours; maintain sterile area

Hypertension

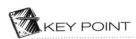 KEY POINT

Elevated pressure of 140/90 mm Hg or greater on 3 consecutive visits.

Data Collection

- Early signs and symptoms: none.
- Late signs and symptoms: nosebleed, headache, visual disturbances, and dizziness.

Management

- Risk factors:
    Modifiable: diet, weight, cholesterol, smoking, oral contraceptives, lifestyle (personality).
    Nonmodifiable: age, sex, family history, race, diabetes.
- Management includes modifying lifestyle prior to introduction of diurectics, antihypertensives, and vasodilators.
- Diet modification: 2-gram sodium restriction (no added salt); decrease cholesterol intake and attempt to maintain cholesterol at a serum level of less than 200 mg/dL.
- Avoid oral contraceptives.
- Smoking cessation.
- Alcohol restriction to less than one ounce per day.
- Reduce weight.
- Increase activity with aerobic exercise.
- Medications: antihypertensives, vasodilators, and diuretics.

Thrombophlebitis—Deep Vein Thrombosis (DVT)

Data Collection

- Signs and symptoms include calf pain, redness, warmth to the touch over area, leg circumference larger in the affected leg (extremity), and positive Homan's sign (pain upon dorsiflexion of foot).
- Major complication is potential for a pulmonary embolism.

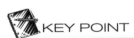 KEY POINT

If any client complains of restlessness, shortness of breath, or chest pain consider pulmonary embolism.

- To prevent the formation of DVTs in those at risk, the physician may order subcutaneous injection of heparin (in abdomen).

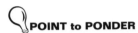

POINT to PONDER

Teach for diet and selection of foods: pick fresh first, then frozen, but avoid canned. Avoid prepared foods and take-out foods.

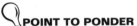

POINT TO PONDER

Look for the problem in clients who are in postoperative recovery process, on bedrest, have spinal cord injury, are obese, taking oral contraceptives, or recovering from CHF.

- Early activity/ambulation and isometric exercise of legs while in bed.
- The use of Venodyne or pneumo boots postoperatively is recommended.

Management After DVT Occurs

- Elevate foot of bed by 6 inches.
- Check for bleeding and institute bleeding precautions.

▶ SAFETY TIP

Heparin will be started IV, so make sure no aspirin products are being taken.

Monitor PTT or APTT (remember two t's [tt] make an H)

Buerger's Disease (Thromboangiitis)

◀ **Arterial Disorders**

Data Collection

- Signs and symptoms include pain (including rest pain); claudication; and red toes with edema and cyanosis in advanced stages, which can lead to ulcerations and gangrene of the toes.

Management

- Stop smoking, keep extremities warm, do not cross legs when sitting, elevate head of bed, place padding between toes, maintain nail care, and do not elevate feet.

Raynaud's Disease

- Incidence is greater in females between 15 and 45 years of age.
- Occurs in response to cold temperatures.

Data Collection

- Signs and symptoms include bilateral pallor of hands/extremities, which proceeds to cyanosis, and then to rubor with pain.

Management

- Keep the extremities warm by avoiding refrigerators and freezers to limit episodes of vasoconstriction. Discourage smoking and utilize cardiovascular risk factor management.

Anatomy, Physiology, ▶
and Pathophysiology

Thorax

- Ribs: 12 pairs total (11 and 12 are floating ribs).
- Sternum: manubrium, body, xiphoid process
- Scapula lies posteriorly from T1 (top) to T7 (bottom).

Chest Deformities

Scoliosis	Lateral deviation which may be seen in children.
Kyphosis	Hunched-over appearance caused by collapse of vertebrae, usually seen in older adults with osteoporosis.
Kyphoscoliosis	The combination of both lateral and thoracic deviations.
Lordosis	Disease of hips or lumbar vertebrae resulting in a flat appearance of lumbar area.
Barrel chest	Enlarged diameter of the chest noted in pulmonary emphysema, and seen in newborns.
Flail chest	Seen in severe trauma cases.

Airways

- Trachea: major entry airway to lungs.
- Main stem bronchus (right and left) divide at the bottom of the trachea; right main stem bronchus is "straighter" than the left and creates a greater possibility for aspiration pneumonia on right side.

Lungs

- Right lung has three lobes and left lung two lobes.
- Alveoli are grape-like air sacs that exchange oxygen and carbon dioxide; destruction of large numbers can result in emphysema.

Breathing Patterns

- Adult: normal rate is between 10 to 18 breaths per minute.
- Newborn: 44 breaths per minute.
- Bradypnea: a decreased rate of breathing that can occur in conditions such as coma or other brain injury and alcohol or drug overdose.
- Tachypnea: an increased rate of breathing caused by problems such as anxiety, exercise, fever, pain, cardiac disease, or anemia.
- Cheyne–Stokes: cycles of breathing with rapid periods followed by periods of apnea; can occur in neurologic dysfunction such as coma, increased intracranial pressure, and cerebral hypoxia, and is a grave sign.
- Dyspnea: shortness of breath or difficulty breathing experienced by persons with chronic lung disease or who have participated in heavy exercise.
- Orthopnea: inability to breathe while lying flat; occurs in CHF, cardiac disease, and pulmonary edema.
- Stridor: crowing sound of respiration which indicates an acute narrowing of airway such as seen in croup or asthma.
- Crackles (rales): bubbling or crackling sounds heard in the lung fields and appearing in conditions such as pneumonias, consolida-

tions, CHF (bilateral lung fields), prolonged bedrest (clear on cough), and acute episodes of bronchitis and COPD.

- Wheezes: musical sounds created by a narrowed bronchial airway in conditions such as COPD (especially in asthma), and foreign body obstruction.

POINT TO PONDER

Caution: Disappearance of a wheeze in acute conditions indicates airway obstruction (emergency).

Sputum Production

Greenish color	Acute bronchitis, lung abscess, pneumonias, tuberculosis.
Whitish color	Asthma, chronic bronchitis.
Red color	Bronchogenic carcinoma or tuberculosis.
Pink and frothy	Congestive heart failure and pulmonary edema.

Disturbances in Oxygen and Carbon Dioxide Exchange

- Respiratory acidosis: caused by respiratory insufficiency, respiratory arrest, airway obstruction, COPD.
    Client will have change in level of consciousness such as confusion, lethargy, drowsiness, headache, and rapid breathing.
- Respiratory alkalosis: caused by hyperventilation from pain, anxiety, and severe thyroid disease.
    Client will have tingling and numbness, lightheadedness, and change in level of consciousness (may faint or lapse into a coma).
- Metabolic acidosis: caused by renal failure, diabetic ketoacidosis, and diarrhea.
    Client will have deep and rapid respirations (Kussmaul's breathing), confusion, and coma.
- Metabolic alkalosis: caused by vomiting, nasogastric suction, taking too much antacid with sodium bicarbonate.
    Client will have decreased respiratory rate, confusion, increased muscle irritability and twitching, and seizures.

Chest x-ray

- Performed in x-ray department or at bedside

CLINICAL NURSING IMPLICATIONS

- Make sure all jewelry is off and IV tubing is away from the client. If a nurse must hold the client, he or she should wear a lead shield and, if pregnant, not be present at all. Chest x-rays can be used to identify changes of the lungs and thorax.
- Most common findings are pneumonia, atelectasis, and pneumothorax.

Coughing and Deep Breathing, and Postural Drainage

- Encourage postoperative clients and clients with lung diseases such as pneumonia or atelectasis to breathe deeply 10 times per hour when awake after surgical procedures; may use incentive spirometer as well, if ordered.
- Frequent position changes will help to drain secretions from the parts of the lung that have fluid and consolidation. (The area of the lung to be drained should be above other parts of the chest with client lying on opposite side.) Allow gravity to drain area. Do not

◀ **Data Collection, Procedures, and Treatments**

place clients with increased intracranial pressure in Trendelenburg position (head down–feet up).

- Contraindications for postural drainage include chest injuries, bleeding disorders, severe osteoporosis, rib fractures, and sometimes after V-P shunt placement.

Sputum Collection

Respiratory Cultures

- Early morning specimen is best collected in a sterile cup.
- Obtained for culture and sensitivity, cytology (cell types), and acid-fast bacillus (AFB) (tuberculosis).
- Check for a valid physician order.
- Properly identify the client and teach the client how to raise sputum.
- Provide the client with a specimen container the night before.
- Do not let the client eat or drink anything (except water), brush teeth, or wash mouth out with rinses or mouthwashes before obtaining sample.

Oxygen Delivery Systems

- Use if ordered by physician, assess the client before use, and place no smoking signs at room. Instruct client not to smoke.

Nasal Cannula

- Assess nares every 8 hours.
- Apply water soluble lubricant to nose to prevent irritation.
- Delivers low flow levels of 24 to 40%.
- Select for those with COPD/hypoxic drive who need low-flow oxygen at 2 to 3 liters per minute.
- Can deliver up to 6 liters per minute.

Face Mask

- Short-term usage.
- Delivers flow levels of 30 to 60% oxygen.
- Delivers 4 to 6 liters per minute.
- Good for use in emergency situations.

Mask With a Rebreathing Bag

- Delivers higher concentrations of oxygen (90 to 100%).
- Check to make sure bag is full of air.

Venturi Mask and Nonrebreathing System

- Very accurate oxygen delivery from 24 to 45% (up to 60 to 100%).

Suctioning

- Verify the physician order.
- Obtain a baseline (presuction) assessment including ability to breathe, pulse, respiration rate, and blood pressure.
- Encourage clients to cough up/remove secretions on their own.
- Splint chest if necessary to encourage cough.
- Explain procedure.
- For best effect in oral suctioning to improve airway access, move the conscious client into the semi-Fowler's position, and the unconscious client onto his or her side.
- Set wall suction pressure at 60 to 100 mm Hg for adults and 50 to 90 mm Hg for infants.
- For tracheal or oral suctioning, lubricate the catheter with sterile H_2O; for nasal suctioning, lubricate the catheter with a water-soluble lubricant.
- In order to thin out thick (tenacious) sputum in trachea, instill 3 to 5 mL of sterile H_2O into tracheostomy tube to loosen secretions.
- Place sterile glove on dominant hand.
- Apply suction no longer than 10 seconds, and suction only during withdrawal of catheter.
- Prior to suctioning the client with a tracheostomy, preoxygenate with 100% O_2, 3 to 5 breaths via Ambu bag.
- Allow at least 20 seconds between suctioning passes, and ventilate the tracheostomy client with 3 to 5 breaths between passes.
- Suction from least to most contaminated by suctioning tracheostomy first, mouth second, and nose third.

▶ SAFETY TIP

Always wear glasses/goggles to suction, and wear mask for communicable diseases with airborne transmission.

Tracheostomy Care

- Assemble equipment and explain procedure to client.
- Cleaning solution: H_2O_2 and normal sterile saline, followed by a normal saline rinse which is used to clean inner cannula in a sterile basin after removal.
- Use tracheostomy dressings only (no cut 4 x 4s).
- Tie all ties with a square knot, and never cut old ties until new ties are in place.
- Tracheostomy cuffs are low-pressure cuffs having no more than 15 to 20 mm Hg of pressure in them.
- Fenestrated tracheostomy tube used for speech.

POINT TO PONDER

Emergency equipment at bedside for tracheostomy client: extra tracheostomy set, Kelly clamps, and suction machine.

Chest Tubes

- Designed to remove air or secretions (upper for air and lower for secretions) and used after pneumothorax or chest surgery (lobectomy) to reexpand lung.

- **Not** used for pneumonectomy (lung removal).

- If accidental disconnection of the chest tube and the container occurs, place end of chest tube in bottle with 2 cm of sterile water or clamp tube close to client. Then wipe end of chest tube and drainage tube with an iodine-based disinfectant and reconnect. Report to nursing supervisor or physician immediately.

- Pleur-evac/3-chamber/3-bottle suction:
  Suction control chamber/bottle closest to suction.
  Water seal chamber/bottle is middle seal.
  Drainage collection chamber/bottle closest to tube.

- Suction control chamber/bottle regulated at −15 to −20 cm H_2O (per order of physician. Pleur-evac is controlled by the amount of water in the suction control chamber).

- Suction control chamber *should bubble* regularly when suction is being utilized.

- Water seal chamber is filled to premeasured level and *should not bubble,* but level of water in the chamber will fluctuate with respiration.

- Drainage chamber collects blood/secretions. Notify supervisor or physician if secretions are greater than 100 mL per hour.

- Troubleshooting: If the nurse encounters any of the following, he or she should report immediately to charge nurse or supervisor.
  Problem: Suction control chamber is not bubbling.
    Check amount of suction at wall (to see if it is on), check connections between suction control chamber/bottle and wall, and check tubing for kinks.
  Problem: Water seal chamber/bottle is bubbling.
    Check for a leak in connections from drainage collection chamber/bottle to client, tape all connections, and recheck for continued bubbling.
  Problem: Water seal chamber bubbles when client coughs.
    Check for leaks in connections as above.
  Problem: Water seal chamber not fluctuating with respirations.
    Tube from client to collection chamber/bottle is blocked or kinked, or lung has reexpanded.

► SAFETY TIPS

Always keep entire system below the level of the lung.

Keep 6-foot flexible tube connecting chest tube to Pleur-evac from kinking or hanging too low.

When transporting client, keep system closed.

For emergency, keep two clamps, tape, and suction at bedside.

When removal of tube performed by surgeon, teach client to take a deep breath and exhale completely. Tube removed during deep exhalation and dressing applied immediately to avoid leaks.

Bronchoscopy

Preprocedurally

- Ensure that the client is NPO for 8 hours prior to procedure.
- Send client with chart and all signed permissions.

Postprocedurally

- Obtain vital signs every 15 minutes until stable (for at least one hour).
- Observe for bleeding/signs of shock.

Pulmonary Function Studies (PFTs)

- Used to assess the client's ability to move air in and out of the lungs. Will change in lung disorders such as emphysema and other chronic lung diseases. Client will blow into a tube connected to a pulmonary function device to measure the lung capacity and amount of air exhaled.

Blood Test

Serum Aminophylline (Theophylline) Level

- Normal: 5 to 20 μg/mL for therapeutic effect.

CLINICAL NURSING IMPLICATIONS:

- Note signs and symptoms of toxicity including nausea, vomiting, seizures, insomnia, and restlessness. Client should be monitored every 6 to 12 months once stabilized.

Pneumonia

- Some examples of organisms causing pneumonia include pneumococcal, viral, *Mycoplasma pneumoniae, Legionella pneumophila* (Legionnaire's disease), and pneumocystis carinii pneumonia (PCP).
- Nosocomial pneumonias (known as hospital acquired) include *Klebsiella, Pseudomonas,* aspiration, and staphylococcal.

Management

- Recommend that all elderly, disabled, and respiratory-impaired individuals get the pneumococcal and influenza vaccines.
- When caring for the client raising sputum, have airway and suction readily available.
- Position in semi-Fowler's position to improve airway opening and improve breathing.

POINT TO PONDER

NPO until return of gag reflex.

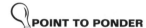 **Respiratory Disorders**

POINT TO PONDER

Handwashing is the key to limiting spread of all infections, especially with respiratory agents.

- Encourage coughing and deep breathing or incentive spirometry every hour if ordered.
- Push fluids to 3 liters per day.
- Give antibiotics to treat specific organisms.
- Administer oxygen as ordered.

Tuberculosis

- Pulmonary tuberculosis spread by airborne droplet nuclei.
- Risk factors: old age, recent immigration, overcrowded conditions, and AIDS clients
- BCG (Bacille Calmette-Guérin) vaccine:
  Used in areas with high incidence of TB.
  Client will have positive reaction with a purified protein derivative (PPD).
- TB test:
  Mantoux (PPD): intradermal read in 48 to 72 hours
  5 Tuberculin units
- Mantoux positive if area is 10 mm indurated (raised) and red or more. *Exception:* Immunosuppressed clients such as those with AIDS are considered positive with 5-mm indurated area.

▶ SAFETY TIP

Use a 25-gauge needle and keep bevel up while placing the syringe at a 15-degree angle for the injection. Do not rub after injection of solution.

- Sputum sample obtained for acid-fast bacilli (AFB) is considered positive for disease when the AFB *grow* in culture.
- Nutrition: high-calorie, high-protein diet with supplements.
- Medication compliance major is the biggest teaching point.
- Medication for prophylactic treatment or treatment of new converter is isoniazid (INH).
- Pyridoxine (vitamin B_6) for side effects of INH, which include peripheral neuropathy.
- Multiple drugs taken for active disease, including rifampin, ethambutal, streptomycin, and INH.

Pulmonary Embolism

- Risk factor: postoperative inactivity/bedrest or history of deep vein thrombosis (DVT).

Management

- Sit client up in high-Fowler's position.
- Administer oxygen as ordered.

POINT TO PONDER

Early symptoms: weight loss, anorexia, fatigue, fever.
Later symptoms: cough, sputum production, night sweats.

POINT TO PONDER

If ordered, encourage patient to take medications for at least 9 months.

- Stay with client.
- Call for help.
- Prepare for surgery.
- Monitor vital signs every 15 minutes until stable.

Chronic Obstructive Pulmonary Disease

- Three types:
   Asthma: increased mucus production and spasm.
   Bronchitis: cough for 3 months in 2 consecutive years ("blue bloater").
   Emphysema: shortness of breath with increased A-P (anterior–posterior) diameter ("pink puffer").
- Other signs and symptoms of advanced disease include fatigue, orthopnea (with heart failure/cor pulmonale), cyanosis (bronchitis), and reddish/ruddy color (emphysema).

Management Issues

- Administer the following with a physician order:
   Low-flow oxygen (2 L/min). Remember, because of *hypoxic drive*, high doses of oxygen are contraindicated. Question all orders for high-flow oxygen in these clients.
- Teach client about pursed-lip breathing.
- Encourage cough and deep breathing with postural drainage during acute exacerbations of the problem.
- Avoid postural drainage one hour before and one hour after meals to prevent loss of appetite before and vomiting after meals.
- The recommendation of *6 small meals per day* (with supplements) will improve the nutritional status and encourage the intake of 3 liters of fluid per day (unless history of heart failure).
- Encourage communication between family and client regarding everyday management.
- Compliance major issue:
   Medications, smoking, staying away from crowds, and diet.
- The type and color of sputum produced by client is whitish to pale yellow color. Teach client to report any green sputum or change in color, as it usually means they are experiencing an acute infection.

▶ SAFETY TIP

Keep client away from anyone with respiratory infections, crowds, smokers, or using any type of powders.

- Watch for stomach disorders/complaints when taking bronchodilating drugs (potential for ulcers). The physician may suggest antacids to eliminate ulcer potential.

POINT TO PONDER

Signs and symptoms of P.E.:
   Early: anxiety and restlessness.
   Late: sudden dsypnea, nonproductive cough, tachycardia.

POINT TO PONDER

Early signs and symptoms:
   Gradual progressive shortness of breath (emphysema).
   Early morning (smoker's) cough (bronchitis).
Classic signs and symptoms:
   Cough, wheezing and dyspnea (gradual).

Pneumothorax

Data Collection

- Subjective: Client complains of sudden onset of shortness of breath and chest pain.
- Objective: Client presents with dyspnea, cyanosis, tachycardia, and hypotension. May have rib deformity after injury, which can lead to decreased movement of the affected side of the chest.

Emergency Management

- Stay with client.
- Call for help.
- Sit client up in high-Fowler's position.
- Will usually require insertion of chest tube by physician.

Acute Respiratory Failure

Early Signs and Symptoms

- Restlessness, anxiety, tachycardia.

Late Signs and Symptoms

- Tachypnea, cardiac irregularities, changes in level of consciousness including confusion, lethargy, stupor, or coma.

Management of Acute Respiratory Failure

- *Airway, Breathing, Circulation, Safety*
- *Airway:*
  Extend neck; don't hyperextend.
  Have airways available.
  Have suction available.
- *Breathing:*
  Administer humidified oxygen per order.
  Position in high-Fowler's position if awake and flat if unconscious.
  Monitor efforts to breathe and potential airway obstruction.
- *Circulation:*
  Monitor vital signs every 15 minutes.
  Note irregularities of heart rate and rhythm.
- *Safety:*
  Never leave the client who is experiencing respiratory difficulty.

Tracheostomy Surgery (may include a radical neck dissection)

- Performed for laryngeal carcinoma.

► SAFETY TIPS

Airway: tracheostomy care and management to maintain patent airway.

Breathing: assess breathing pattern every two hours.

Circulation: observe for bleeding. Assess for signs of swelling, airway narrowing, and vital signs changes of impending shock. Normal blood/drainage amount 100 mL in first 24 hours.

Erythrocytes

- Red blood cells (RBCs) carry oxygen to cells and remove CO_2 back to lungs. Average life span is 120 days. Hemoglobin is the iron component of RBCs that picks up oxygen.

Leukocytes

- White blood cells (WBCs) increase in response to infections and inflammation.

    Neutrophils = respond to **bacterial infection.**
    Lymphocytes = respond to **infection,** usually **viral.**

Complete Blood Count (CBC) (Venipuncture)

- Measures RBCs, hemoglobin, WBCs, and a differential of the types of WBCs.

- Key points in collection: Get medication history (anticoagulants and aspirin will affect coagulation tests for up to 7 to 14 days); applying the tourniquet for too long a period will alter the results of many blood tests. Universal precautions required.

RBC Count

- Normal: adult, 4.6 to 6.0×10^{12}; child, 3.8 to 5.5×10^{12}.

Clinical Nursing Implications

- Too few RBCs indicate anemia or blood loss.
- Too many indicate polycythemia or dehydration.

Hematocrit (Percentage of Cells in Plasma)

- Normal: adult female, 37 to 48%; adult male, 45 to 52%; child, 1 to 3 years, 29 to 40%; child, 4 to 10 years, 31 to 43%.

Clinical Nursing Implications

- A low percentage indicates anemia; a high percentage indicates dehydration or polycythemia.

Hemoglobin

- Normal: female, 12 to 16 g/dL; male, 13 to 18 g/dL; child 6 months to 1 year, 10 to 15 g/dL; child 5 to 14 years, 11 to 16 g/dL.

Nursing Implications

- Low levels indicate anemia or acute blood loss.
- High levels are associated with polycythemia or dehydration.

WBC Count

- Normal: adult, 4500 to 10,000 µL; child, 2 years, 6000 to 17,000 µL.

◄ Anatomy, Physiology, and Pathophysiology

◄ Data Collection, Procedures, and Treatments

POINT TO PONDER

Low levels in clients with iron deficiency, poor nutrition, and recent hemorrhage. Elevated levels occur in dehydrated clients with fever and in clients with chronic obstructive pulmonary disease (COPD).

Hematologic System

Increased in acute infections or inflammatory conditions (any -itis condition), myocardial infarction (MI) clients, antibiotic use (the -mycins), and some leukemias. Decreased in AIDS, anemias, some leukemias, and with some medications.

POINT TO PONDER

Clients with low platelet levels should be placed on bleeding precautions, including shaving with electric razors only, no raw fruit or vegetables, minimal injections, pressure over injection sites for at least 5 minutes, and checking stool frequently for occult blood.

Clinical Nursing Implications

- An increase occurs in infection, inflammation, or medication reactions.
- A decrease occurs with immunologic disturbances, severe anemias, or medication reactions.

Platelet Count

- Normal: adult, 150,000 to 400,000 µL; child, 100,000 to 300,000 µL.

Clinical Nursing Implications

- Decreased counts occur in leukemias, liver disease, DIC (disseminated intravascular coagulopathy), and kidney disease.
- Increased counts occur in infections, acute blood loss, or splenectomy.

Blood Transfusions

- Blood is screened for the following: ABO type, Rh factor, VDRL, Coombs' test, hepatitis B and C, human immunodeficiency virus (HIV), human T-lymphotrophic virus (HTLV), and alanine transaminase (ALT).
- Type and crossmatch: Unit is matched against blood from the recipient.
- ABO grouping of blood: If not done correctly, the wrong antigen of blood will be given; this could create renal failure or death from hemolytic reactions.

Transfusion Reactions

Hemolytic Reaction (most serious resulting from incompatibility)

- What to look for:
  Reaction occurs within the first 15 minutes; client will complain of burning along the vein, chest pain or tightness, tachycardia, chills, fever, nausea, vomiting, crackles and wheezes upon auscultation.

- What to do with R.N.:
  Stop transfusion immediately.
  Infuse normal saline at a rate of 1 mL per minute.
  Obtain vital signs.
  Notify physician.
  Obtain blood sample from a distant vein (opposite side).
  Begin oxygen, per order.
  Have epinephrine available.
  Push fluids.
  Obtain urine sample and check for hemoglobinuria.
  Send blood back to blood bank.
  Prepare to administer mannitol if ordered (used to increase diuresis and to prevent or limit acute tubular necrosis).

Allergic Reaction (most common type of reaction)

■ What to look for:

Pruritus; rash; facial redness or edema; complaints of difficulty breathing, tongue swelling, or throat closing; tachycardia; other evidence of anaphylactic reaction.

■ What to do with R.N.:

Stop transfusion immediately.
Infuse normal saline at a rate of 1 mL per minute.
Obtain vital signs.
Notify physician.
Begin oxygen, per order.
Have epinephrine and diphenhydramine hydrochloride (Benadryl) available.
Airway is top priority; prepare for anaphylactic reaction.
Send blood back to blood bank.

Bacterial Reaction (usually occurs later in transfusion)

■ What to look for:

Fever, chills, tachycardia, hypotension, vomiting, abdominal pain, bloody diarrhea.

■ What to do with R.N.:

Stop transfusion immediately.
Infuse normal saline at a rate of 1 mL per minute.
Obtain vital signs.
Notify physician.
Send blood back to blood bank.
Send client blood sample to laboratory.
Prepare for administration of antibiotics.

Circulatory Overload (cardiac reaction to too much fluid)

■ What to look for:

Shortness of breath, nonproductive cough, chest tightness or pain, crackles upon auscultation, and evidence of CHF or pulmonary edema.

■ What to do with R.N.:

Stop transfusion.
Sit the client up and dangle legs over side of bed.
Obtain vital signs.
Notify physician.
Prepare to treat for pulmonary edema, including use of rotating tourniquets, diuretics, and digoxin.

▶ SAFETY TIP

Autologous transfusions are safest because they are the client's own blood; eliminates fear of AIDS transmission.

Jehovah's witnesses cannot have blood transfusions in any form.

Hematologic System

61

Hematologic Disorders ▶ **Anemia**

Acute Blood Loss

- Complaints such as confusion, weakness, lightheadedness, tachycardia, and tachypnea are related to lack of oxygen transfer to cells.
- Managed by stopping hemorrhage and replacing blood lost.

Iron Deficiency

- Complaints are related to blood loss and include weakness, lethargy, dyspnea, tachycardia, pale mucous membranes, dysphasia (Plummer–Vinson syndrome), tarry stools, and pica (especially in young children and during pregnancy).
- Managed by identifying source of chronic blood loss (check stools for occult blood), improving dietary intake, and giving supplemental iron if ordered by physician.
- Assessing the client on iron:
    Vitamin C will improve absorption.
    Ascorbic acid (vitamin C) or juices high in it are often recommended to take iron with.
    If liquid is given, use a straw to avoid staining teeth.
    Stools will become dark and tarry after iron has been started.
    Assess clients taking iron for constipation. Physician may order a stool softener to manage.
    Iron given IM requires the Z-track technique to prevent muscle and skin irritation.

Pernicious Anemia (vitamin B$_{12}$ deficiency, macrocytic)

- Complaints include tingling and numbness; loss of position sense; gait abnormalities; red, beefy tongue (glossitis); and general GI complaints.
- Managed by vitamin B$_{12}$ replacement shots every month; diagnosed by Schilling test.

Sickle Cell Anemia (predominantly seen in Black populations)

- Caused by inherited genetic disorder resulting in cell formation of thicker, more rigid cells that have a tendency to block or slow capillary circulation.
- Complaints include infarction, pain, fever, infections, and pale mucous membranes.
- Nursing management requires maintaining appropriate hydration, avoiding dehydration, and preventing infections.

POINTS TO PONDER

Crises are often associated with pain or a throbbing feeling.

During crises children are placed on bedrest.

ENDOCRINE SYSTEM

Anatomy, Physiology, and Pathophysiology ▶

- The endocrine system includes organs and glands such as the
    Adrenal glands
    Pancreas
    Pituitary gland
    Ovaries
    Thymus
    Thyroid gland

Blood Tests

Blood Glucose

- Normal: adult serum and plasma, 70 to 110 mg/dL, whole blood 60 to 100 mg/dL; child (newborn), 30 to 80 mg/dL; child, 60 to 100 mg/dL.

CLINICAL NURSING IMPLICATIONS

- Finger must be clean and dry prior to stick. Finger is stuck on sides but not on tip to minimize pain (tips are overly sensitive to touch and pain). Do not smear blood on strip; allow drop to dry on strip.

Glucose Tolerance Test

CLINICAL NURSING IMPLICATIONS

- Client drinks a glucose drink, and, at intervals of 1 to 4 hours, samples of urine and blood are taken to monitor the reaction.
- Elevations occur in trauma, infection, diabetes mellitus, and stress.

Postprandial Blood Sugar

- Normal: adult, less than 140 mg/dL/2h; child, less than 120 mg/dL/2h.

CLINICAL NURSING IMPLICATIONS

- Blood is drawn 2 hours after a meal.
- Elevated levels indicate possible diabetes mellitus.

Glycosylated Hemoglobin

- Normal: 6 to 8%.

CLINICAL NURSING IMPLICATIONS

- Elevations help determine the level of diet compliance in diabetics.
- Glucose levels can be evaluated over several weeks.

Diabetes Mellitus

◀ Endocrine Disorders

Type I: Insulin-dependent Diabetes Mellitus (IDDM)

- Characteristics:
  Under 30 years of age.
  Weight loss.
  Presents with the 3 Ps.
  Ketones present in urine.

Type II: Noninsulin-dependent Diabetes Mellitus (NIDDM)

- Characteristics:
  Older adult (over 40)
  Obese
  No ketones in urine.
- Diagnostic tests evaluate the amount of sugar in blood at varying intervals such as fasting, and one or two hours after eating.

POINT TO PONDER

Three Ps of diabetes: polyuria, polyphasia, polydipsia.

Management

- Diet: developed via exchange lists as recommended by the American Diabetic Association.
- Medication administration:
  Insulins
  > Regular insulin peaks in 2 to 4 hours and lasts 5 to 7 hours.
  > NPH insulin peaks in 6 to 12 hours and lasts 18 to 28 hours.
  > Ultralente peaks in 18 to 24 hours and lasts 36 hours.

▶ SAFETY TIP

Make sure insulin-dependent diabetics get appropriate snacks in midafternoon and evening. Types of snacks include fruit selection (grapes, pear, apple) and pretzels, three crackers (graham or wheat) or six saltines, with small piece of cheese or 4 ounces of skim milk.

POINT TO PONDER

If client becomes hypoglycemic midmorning, this effect is caused by regular insulin. If client becomes hypoglycemic in late afternoon, this effect is caused by NPH insulin (providing both insulins were injected in the early morning around 8 A.M.).

POINT TO PONDER

Insulin is supplied in U-100 dosage (100 units per mL). Insulin does not need to be refrigerated, but refrigeration will increase the time of storage prior to use.

- Insulin injections usually given in the morning (around 8 A.M.) and in the late afternoon/early evening (around 5 P.M.)
- Regular insulin and NPH insulin can be mixed. Procedure for mixing:
  > Clean both vial tops. Inject the amount of air into NPH insulin vial that will be withdrawn. Inject the amount of air into regular insulin vial that will be withdrawn. Withdraw insulin from the regular insulin vial. Finally, withdraw the amount of insulin from the NPH vial.
- Rotate sites of injection between arms, legs, and abdomen.
- Teach self-administration and demonstrate how to pinch skin to create an area of subcutaneous tissue in which to inject.
- During times of illness when client is NPO or cannot eat, provide normal dosage of insulin and encourage intake of extra liquids, which include sugars in small amounts (several ounces of regular soft drinks and several crackers every hour, for example).
- Oral hypoglycemics include tolazamide, tolbutamide, chlorpropamide, and glyburide, and can cause hypoglycemic symptoms.

Important Client Teaching Points

- Testing of blood sugar.
- Testing urine for glucose and ketones.

Signs and Symptoms of Hypoglycemia and Hyperglycemia

- Hypoglycemia: hunger, weakness, pallor, diaphoresis, anxiety, fatigue, shakiness, irritability, blurred vision, and disorientation.
- Hyperglycemia: 3 Ps of hyperglycemia.

Management of Hypoglycemia

- Give 10 grams of carbohydrate by taking 2 packets of sugar, 4 ounces of orange juice, 2 to 3 hard candies, or 2 teaspoons of honey.
- Notify physician.

Managment of Hyperglycemia

- Give additional insulin coverage per physician order.

Exercise and Impact on Medications

- Will require a lower amount of insulin; client should consult with physician or nurse practitioner.

Complications Associated With Diabetes Mellitus

PERIPHERAL VASCULAR DISEASE

- Foot problems as a result of skin changes and poor circulation can lead to the development of ulcers, gangrene, and amputations.
- Provide meticulous foot care, including keeping area warm and dry. Discourage crossing of legs; encourage well-fitting shoes, white socks, applying lanolin or lubricant to avoid skin dryness, careful daily inspections to look for dryness, abrasions, or ulcerations.

PERIPHERAL NEUROPATHIC DISORDERS (NEUROPATHIES)

- Signs and symptoms include pain, paresthesia, and loss of position sense (proprioception).

KETOACIDOSIS (TYPE I)

- Symptoms and signs include dry, flushed looked; Kussmaul respirations; a fruity odor on breath; and large amount of ketones found in urine.

Cushing's Syndrome

- Complaints may include weight gain, obesity, hyperglycemia, easy bruising, buffalo hump, and mental disturbances.
- Observe and monitor mental status changes.
- Assist with ADLs for fatigue and lethargy.
- Diet for the client should restrict sodium and carbohydrates and replace potassium.

Addison's Disease

- Complaints are nonspecific and include weakness, lethargy, fatigue, and skin bronzing.
- Replacement of adrenocorticotropic hormone (ACTH) with hydrocortisone per physician order.
- Avoid stress as it increases need for response.

POINT TO PONDER

Think SWISS:
- **S** Salt retention
- **W** Water retention
- **I** Infection prone
- **S** Sugar excess
- **S** Sex characteristic changes

POINT TO PONDER

During hot weather and with exercise, advise clients to increase fluid and sodium intake.

Monitor for Addisonian crisis (stress induced):

Dehydration

Fever

Hypotension

Electrolyte imbalances

Hyperthyroidism

■ Complaints include weight loss, anorexia, insomnia, tachycardia, dyspnea, weakness and fatigue, anxiety, tremulousness, irritability, decreased attention span, and polyuria.

■ Surgical removal of thyroid gland may be required.

■ General management includes quiet, nonstimulating environment; management of bulging eyes with eye patches at night and ointments to keep moist.

Hypothyroidism

■ Complaints include lethargy; weight gain; edema, including facial and eyelid edema; slow speech; decreased hair growth and thinning of hair; and memory loss.

■ Managed by gradually increasing thyroid hormone per physician order.

GASTROINTESTINAL SYSTEM

**Anatomy, Physiology, and ►
Pathophysiology**

Mouth

■ Teeth for chewing, tongue for distinguishing tastes.

Esophagus

■ Swallowing accomplished by peristaltic movements.

Stomach

■ Initially stores and breaks down food.

Intestines

■ Peristaltic waves move foods through digestive tract.

Rectum/Anus

■ Storage of stool and area of defecation.

Skin on Abdomen

■ Stretch marks called striae:
Purple, new or caused by Cushing's disease.
Gray/white, old (previous pregnancies/childbirth, weight gain).

Pain

Appendix	Right lower quadrant with rebound tenderness.
Cholecystitis	Right upper quadrant and right shoulder.
Diverticulitis	Left lower quadrant pains.
Pancreatitis	Midepigastric and radiating to back or left shoulder.
Pelvic inflammatory disease (PID)	Bilateral lower quadrants.
Rectal pain	Posterior and associated with tenesmus (painful defecation).

Anorexia

- Loss of appetite associated with anorexia nervosa, cancer/chemotherapy, cancer of stomach or intestines, and liver disease.

Pica

- Craving for specific foods/substances often associated with eating dirt in children and eating paint; seen in lead poisoning and anemias.

Polyphagia

- Increased appetite associated with diabetes, hyperthyroidism, and eating disorders.

Heart Burn/Morning Sickness

- Frequent complaint in pregnancy and often associated with hiatal hernias and anxiety.

Vomiting

- Usually accompanied by nausea. Associated with medication toxicity, gastrointestinal disease, or increased intracranial pressure.

Hematemesis

- Vomiting of blood associated with bleeding peptic ulcers, esophageal varices, cancer of the stomach, and clotting disorders.

Stools

- *Red* blood in stools: ulcerative colitis, hemorrhoids, carcinoma of lower colon or rectum.
- *Occult* blood in stools (guaiac positive): melena, seen as tarry, blackened color associated with upper GI bleeding, lower GI bleeding, gastric ulcers, gastritis, duodenal ulcers.
- Fat in stools (steatorrhea) associated with malabsorption syndrome; pancreatic disease; and, in children, galactose intolerance. Stools are foul-smelling, greasy, and float in water.
- White stools are associated with barium enema.
- Gray-colored stools are associated with gallbladder disorder and liver disease.

Diarrhea

- Loose or watery stools occurring in disorders such as viral gastrointestinal infection, food poisoning, ulcerative colitis, and Crohn's disease.

POINT TO PONDER

Small, frequent, loose stools (almost like leaking of stool) are often indicative of fecal impaction or obstruction.

Data Collection, Procedures, ▶ and Treatments

POINT TO PONDER

Fluid loss via either end of the GI tract leads to low levels of chlorides.

Constipation

- Dry, hard stools which become difficult to evacuate from the bowel. This problem is frequently associated with decreased fluid intake, overuse of enemas and laxatives, intestinal obstruction, fecal impaction, and cancer of the GI tract.

Ascites

- Fluid in abdomen. The navel may protrude outward in moderate ascites and can occur in liver disease, congestive heart failure, or renal disease.

Blood Tests

Serum Chloride

- Normal: adult, 95 to 105 mEq/L; child, 98 to 105 mEq/L.

CLINICAL NURSING IMPLICATIONS

- Increased in metabolic acidosis.
- Low levels occur in response to vomiting, diarrhea, gastric suction, or use of diuretics.

Stool Specimens

- Collected in a bedpan or cup and checked for color, consistency, shape, and odor. Three days of collection are needed for ova and parasite analysis.
- Urine can interfere with growth.

Blood in Stool

CLINICAL NURSING IMPLICATIONS

- Vitamin C, aspirin, iron, and large amounts of red meat prior to test can interfere with results. After positive result, restriction of these items may be done 2 to 3 days prior to retest. Report all clients with positive results.
- Bleeding can indicate early signs of bowel cancer or other types of hidden GI problems, such as peptic ulcers. Tests are routinely performed to detect internal bleeding in clients on anticoagulant therapy.

Endoscopic Procedures

- Used to directly visualize parts of the gastrointestinal tract.

Colonoscopy

- Liquid diet for 24 hours preprocedurally.
- NPO for 8 hours.
- GoLYTELY taken night before to cleanse bowel.

Sigmoidoscopy

- Liquid diet or small amounts of food for previous 24 hours; Fleet enema unless history of renal disease (high sodium content).

GI series

Upper

- NPO for 8 hours; client will be upright but may be placed in various positions. Laxative postprocedurally to prevent constipating effects of barium.

Lower

- Low-residue diet for 48 hours prior; laxatives and bowel preparation may be ordered, NPO for 8 hours (or after midnight if specified). Client will have abdominal cramps during procedure from barium instillation into lower GI tract. Test will take 30 to 45 minutes. To decrease discomfort, have client breathe deeply and slowly.

Cholecystogram (to assess the gallbladder)

- Assess for allergy to shellfish or iodine.
- Client will take dye tablets the evening before the procedure.
- NPO after taking tablets.
- Procedure lasts about 30 minutes.

Rectal Examination

- Client placed in left side-lying position or the Sims' lateral position. Equipment includes rubber glove, lubricant, and direct light source. Examiner should allow anal sphincter to relax prior to gently inserting finger. Used to assess for impacted stool, prostate gland, and masses.

Stool Examination

- Check for ova and parasites (O&P).
- Occult blood indicates chronic blood loss of GI tract in conditions such as cancer of the colon, peptic ulcers, and ulcerative colitis.

> **POINT TO PONDER**
>
> False positives are associated with eating red meats and vitamin C intake. Omit these for 3 to 4 days prior to test.

Tubes

- Gastric tubes: Levin tube, Salem sump tube, Sengstaken–Blakemore tube.
- Intestinal tubes: Miller–Abbott (double-lumen) tube, Cantor (single-lumen) tube.

Potential Complications in the Client Receiving Total Parenteral Nutrition (TPN)

◄ Nutritional Information

Hyperglycemia

- High dextrose content will cause hyperglycemia, which can lead to dehydration through osmotic diuresis.
- To reduce the potential for this problem, the solution rate is gradually increased during the first 24 hours.
- Urine usually tested for glucose QID (small amounts of sugar may be found; report ketones immediately).

> **POINT TO PONDER**
>
> Look for signs and symptoms of hyperglycemia (3 Ps = polydipsia, polyphagia, polyuria).

► SAFETY TIP

If ketones are present or urine reveals 3+ or 4+ sugar, notify physician and dietician.

Pneumothorax

■ If client develops sudden restlessness, anxiety, tachycardia, and dyspnea, assess chest for breath sounds (absent in pneumothorax). No fluid will be started until position of line has been verified by an x-ray.

Air Embolism

■ Signs and symptoms include anxiety, agitation, difficulty breathing, and dyspnea. Position client in Trendelenburg position on left side and notify physician immediately.

Infection

■ Septic infections may develop if aseptic techniques are not followed. Assess client for fever and other signs of infection.

Tube Feedings

■ Tubes are made of plastic or rubber and are usually radiopaque so they can be seen on x-ray.

Tube Types

■ Nasal tubes have a very small bore.
■ Oral tubes have a large bore.
■ Gastrostomy and jejunostomy tubes have large bores.

► SAFETY TIP

Check tube for placement prior to each feeding and every 4 hours when on continuous feeding.

POINT TO PONDER

Whenever stomach contents are aspirated, they should be replaced to prevent metabolic alkalosis.

■ Three methods to check placement of tube:
  1. Most accurate way is x-ray of stomach.
  2. Check via auscultation: inject 10 mL of air into tube while placing stethoscope over area of gastric bubble and listen for rush of air. If heard easily, position is usually correct.
  3. Check via aspiration: aspirate stomach contents and check for pH. A pH of 3.0 is close to stomach acid content.

Hold Feedings

- Feedings should be held when the amount of aspirate (prior to feedings) exceeds 100 mL or if the amount is greater than the amount of one hour of feeding being delivered on a continuous basis. **Action: Hold feeding and recheck within the hour.**
- Weigh all tube-fed clients daily.

► SAFETY TIP

An open can of feeding is good for four to six hours if left unrefrigerated.

Give free water (100 mL) every 4 hours.

Always keep head of bed elevated to prevent aspiration of tube feedings.

Complications, Problems, and Solutions Encountered in Tube Feedings

- To prevent nasal irritation:
  Lubricate nares with water-soluble lubricant (KY jelly) to maintain mucous membranes.
- For vomiting:
  Hold feeding solution and notify supervisor.
  When tube feeding is ordered to be resumed:
  1. Check the feeding solution to make sure it has not gone bad/become contaminated.
  2. Recheck tube placement.
  3. Check the rate and volume of infusion.
  4. Sit client in high-Fowler's position.
  5. Make sure to keep client sitting up for at least 30 minutes after feeding (never lie client flat).

- Understanding food types and examples will assist in making recommendations for clients with dietary problems or need for adjustments. ◄ **Diet Information to Know**

Selected Diet Types

Bland and Fiber Restricted (Low Residue)

- Foods without texture.
- Low residue and low in fiber.
- No seasoning, nuts, grains, seeds, raw vegetables, raw fruits, or potato skins.
- Cooked, strained vegetables, cooked fruits OK.
- Cooked, mashed potatoes OK.

- Sweets such as hard candy, jelly beans OK.
- No nuts, raisins, coconuts.

BRAT

- **B**ananas, **R**ice, **A**pplesauce, and **T**oast.
- Used for children with vomiting and/or diarrhea.

Diabetic

- Content:

Carbohydrates	50%	
Protein	20%	
Fat	30%	

Liquid

- Used postoperatively.
- Progress from NPO to clear liquids, to liquids, to soft, to soft solids, to solids.

Clear Liquid

- Clear fruit juices, Jello, Popsicles, cola, ginger ale, orange soda, clear broths, tea or coffee without milk.

Low Fat/Low Cholesterol

- Chicken without skin, meat with low fat content, vegetables OK, breads OK, skim milk products OK.
- Avoid shrimp, organ meats, fatty meats, eggs with yolks, and baked goods.
- Remember, the three Cs to avoid include **C**ake, **C**ookies, and **C**reams.

Low Sodium

- 2 gram (2000 mg) restriction = no table salt, salt with cooking OK, no processed foods.
- 1 gram (1000 mg) restriction = no salt added to cooking, minimal butter/margarine, no cheeses, no canned vegetables.
- $1/2$ gram (500 mg) restriction = "low"-sodium foods only, milk (1 to 2 cups per day), small amounts of meat.

Foods High in Specific Areas

Foods High in Calcium

- Milk, yogurt, cheddar cheese, pudding, ice cream, cottage cheese, oysters, sardines, salmon, and spinach.

Foods High in Potassium

- Liver, pork, hot dogs, chicken, scallops, avocado, artichokes, asparagus, beans, celery, carrots, kale, leeks, mushrooms, potatoes, spinach, squash, cantaloupes, and honeydew melons.

Foods High in Sodium

- Ham, sausage, dried beef, hot dogs, cheese, olives, sauerkraut, and processed foods.

Foods High in Vitamin A

- Sweet potatoes, broccoli, spinach, kale, lettuce, carrots, squash, and corn.

Foods High in Vitamin C

- Oranges, grapefruits, tomatoes, cabbage, broccoli, cantaloupes, and honeydew melons.

Candidal Infection (Thrush)

◀ **Gastrointestinal Disorders**

Data Collection

- Subjective:
  Client complaints include pain and burning in mouth and throat.
  Client may notice a change in taste of foods or complain of funny taste in mouth.
- Objective:
  Mouth lesions appear as whitish, pale, bluish, and cheesy. Usually occurs in infants and immunosuppressed clients, AIDS clients, steroid overuse, infants, and people suffering from general debility.
- Management:
  Treated with nystatin (antifungal) swish and swallow (as ordered).
  Teach client to avoid hot and cold fluids; give tepid or cool fluids, and offer bland, not spicy, foods.
  May require tube feedings in severe instances when the infection proceeds into the esophagus.

Oral Carcinoma

Data Collection

- Objective:
  Client may have white or dark red patches in the mouth. Especially look for in the person with a history of smoking or heavy alcohol intake.
- Managed with surgery, radiation, and chemotherapy.

Hiatal Hernia

Data Collection

- Symptoms of heartburn, reflux, and dysphasia one to three hours after eating and when in bed.
- Common complaint in the elderly.

Management

- Elevate head of bed with blocks 4 to 6 inches off floor.

POINT TO PONDER

Teach client to not eat within 3 hours before bedtime.

- Maintain a low-fat diet that avoids tea, coffee, alcohol, fruit juices, and spicy foods.
- Offer small, frequent meals (4 to 6 per day).
- Antacids may help in relieving heartburn.

Peptic Ulcer Disease (PUD)

Data Collection

Type	Pain	What to Do
Gastric	1/2 to 1 hour after eating Not relieved with food May have nausea and vomiting	Antacids help
Duodenal	Intermittent pain Relieved with food Awakens client at 2 A.M.	Antacids help, food helps decrease pain

- Client should avoid spices, hot liquids, and caffeine-based drinks.
- The client with a gastric ulcer will not want to eat, and the person with a duodenal ulcer gets relief from eating.

POINT TO PONDER

Starve a gastric ulcer and feed a duodenal ulcer.

Gastric Resection (to treat ulcers and cancer of stomach)

- Procedures: Billroth I or II, subtotal gastrectomy, total gastrectomy, vagotomy.

Data Collection for Postoperative Complications

- Hemorrhage:
  Observe for red drainage postoperatively in nasogastric (NG) suction; monitor vital signs and signs and symptoms of impending shock
- Dumping syndrome:
  Symptoms: weakness, dizziness, fainting, diaphoresis, and hypotension.
- Peritonitis:
  Leakage of stomach contents at incision site will allow material to enter peritoneal cavity, resulting in pain and infection.

POINT TO PONDER

Nasogastric suction helps reduce nausea and vomiting in all types of clients. Low NG suction reduces pressure on structure site.

Chronic Inflammatory Bowel Disease

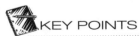

KEY POINTS

Ulcerative colitis: middle-aged adult, bloody, liquid, diarrhea with 15 to 20 loose stools per day with diffuse pain.

Crohn's disease: teenager/young adult with diarrhea of 10 to 15 loose stools per day without bleeding. Stools are usually foul smelling, and pain is reported in the right lower quadrant.

- Management includes controlling diarrhea, relieving pain, and improving nutritional intake with TPN.

Obstruction

- Types: volvulus, intussusception, adhesions, tumors.
- Assess history for surgery, diet, and family history for past GI disorders.
- Signs and symptoms include constipation, abdominal distention, abdominal pain, nausea, and vomiting

Ostomies

Type	Stool	Irrigation	Regulation
Ileostomy	Liquid	No irrigation	No regulation
Asending colostomy	Soft/liquid	No irrigation	No regulation
Transverse colostomy	Soft	No irrigation	No regulation
Sigmoid colostomy	Formed	Irrigation OK	Can be regulated

- Nursing management includes maintaining skin integrity and fluid balance, and helping the client adapt to body image changes.
- The normal stoma color is pink. Report any changes such as cyanosis, duskiness, and blackened, brownish, or pale mucosa.
- Initially stoma should protrude slightly (1 inch) outward, which will decrease when edema resolves.
- Ostomy should begin functioning within 48 hours postoperatively.
- Client should avoid gas-forming foods, including cabbage, onions, beans, eggs, broccoli, asparagus, and beer and other alcohol.

Hepatitis

Type	Route of Infection	Incubation Period
Type A	Fecal–oral	15 to 45 days (short)
Type B	Blood and secretions	30 to 160 days (long)
Type C	Blood and secretions	50 days (intermediate)

- Source of spread: Type A, fecal–oral; types B and C, parenteral and bloodborne.
- Universal precautions are effective in preventing spread of all forms.
- Vaccine available for hepatitis B is given as a course of three different injections, including an initial injection followed by another in 1 month and another in 6 months.

Liver Disease and Cirrhosis

Data Collection

- Subjective and objective findings:
    Early complaints of liver disease include anorexia, nausea, vomiting, diarrhea, clay-colored stools, and lethargy.
    Late findings include handwriting changes, tremor, confusion, asterixis (obvious tremor), enlarged liver, ascites (check and record abdominal girth), fruity odor of breath, and coma.

POINT TO PONDER

Persons at risk for type A hepatitis: day care workers, international travelers, and people in prisons and developmentally disabled homes. Persons at risk for type B hepatitis: health care workers, hemodialysis patients, blood transfusion patients, intravenous drug abusers, those who practice high-risk sexual behaviors, and prison populations.

General Management

- Restrict protein to 40 to 50 g/day with sodium restriction.
- Weigh daily.
- Avoid constipation.
- Check stools for occult blood.
- No analgesics, sedatives, or narcotics allowed.
- Observe for bleeding.

Complications of Advanced Liver Disease

- Esophageal varices:
    Client presents with hematemesis (vomiting blood) and a shock-like condition. Major medical emergency related to shock.
- Encephalopathy:
    Reduce ammonia levels by administering medications per order (lactulose or neomycin per order).
    Diet should be low/moderate protein (40 g/day) and high calories (more than 1500 per day).
    Fluid restriction 1500 mL; diuretics as ordered (watch for electrolyte imbalances).

Cholelithiasis (gallstones)

Data Collection

- Pain is steady, severe, and colicky, accompanied by nausea and vomiting, with right upper quadrant tenderness.
- Managed with a low-fat diet and vitamin supplements.

POINT TO PONDER

Morphine sulfate is contraindicated in patients with gallbladder disease.

GENITOURINARY SYSTEM

Anatomy, Physiology, ▶ and Pathophysiology

Kidneys

- The organs which remove waste from the bloodstream, help to stimulate new RBCs, and maintain fluid and electrolyte balance.

Ureters

- Smooth muscle tubes that allow urine to flow away from the kidneys.

Bladder

- Stores urine before voiding.

Urethra

- Begins in bladder and drains urine to the outside of body.
- The female urethra is between 2 and 4 cm in length.
- The male urethra is between 18 and 20 cm in length.

Complaints

Pain

- *Urethral pain* is usually described as a burning feeling.

POINT TO PONDER

Women are more likely to have urinary tract infections because of the shortened length of the urethra and its close proximity to the anus.

- *Bladder pain* is usually felt in the lower abdomen.
- *Ureteral* pain occurs with obstruction and is often described as a sharp pain radiating down into the groin and back.
- *Kidney pain* is usually felt in the back but can radiate into the pelvic area and the testes.

Dysuria

- Pain during urination that often indicates infections.

Frequency

- Clients complain of urinating often, which can mean the bladder is irritated or infected.

Hematuria

- Frank blood in the urine occurs as a result of trauma or tumor. Occult blood in the urine may indicate bleeding disorder, urinary tract infection, or inflammation.

Oliguria/Anuria

- A decreased urine output or absent urine output may be caused by obstruction in outflow, renal failure, shock, or trauma.

Blood Tests

Serum Blood Urea Nitrogen (BUN)

- Normal: adult, 5 to 25 mg/dL; child, 5 to 20 mg/dL.

CLINICAL NURSING IMPLICATIONS

- Elevation indicates diseased kidney or dehydration and nephrotoxic reactions to some medications (the *-mycins*).
- Decreased levels can be caused by overhydration, an increase in antidiuretic hormone secretion, or pregnancy.

Serum Creatinine

- Normal: adult, 0.5 to 1.5 mg/dL; child, 0.4 to 1.2 mg/dL.

CLINICAL NURSING IMPLICATIONS

- Increased levels indicate renal dysfunction.
- Decreased levels are uncommon.

Serum Calcium

- Normal: adult, 9 to 11 mg/dL; child, 9 to 11.5 mg/dL.

CLINICAL NURSING IMPLICATIONS

- Decreased levels indicate severe renal disease or failure, severe malnutrition, or osteoporosis (but may be normal if calcium is released from bones and teeth). Increased levels are related to hyperparathyroidism, bone disease, tumors, thiazide diuretics, dehydration, or excessive milk intake.

◄ **Data Collection, Procedures, and Treatments**

Serum Phosphorus

- Normal: adult, 2.5 to 4.5 mg/dL; child, 4.5 to 5.5 mg/dL.

CLINICAL NURSING IMPLICATIONS

- Must be sent to the lab quickly.
- Increased levels can indicate hypothyroidism, renal failure, or possible malignancy.
- Decreased levels are observed in hypercalcemia, diuretic use, malabsorption syndrome, and alcohol withdrawal.

Serum Magnesium

- Normal: adult, 1.5 to 2.5 mEq/L; child, 1.6 to 2.6 mEq/L.

CLINICAL NURSING IMPLICATIONS

- Increased levels are associated with renal failure, diabetes mellitus, or dehydration.
- Decreased levels are associated with chronic nutritional problems such as alcoholism, use of diuretics, and some antibiotics.

Routine Urinalysis

- Requires a minimum of 10 mL urine.
- Routine urine tests are often performed on admission or at time of physical to detect infections, dehydration, diabetes, and numerous other problems.

Specific Gravity

- Normal: 1.005 to 1.030.

CLINICAL NURSING IMPLICATIONS

- High specific gravity can occur if glucose, protein, or dye is in the urine.
- High specific gravity usually signifies lack of fluid (concentrated urine) as is seen in dehydration.
- Decreased (low specific gravity) can be indicative of diabetes insipidus or can occur with intake of large volumes of water.

Color

- Normal ranges from straw to amber.

CLINICAL NURSING IMPLICATIONS

- Discoloration occurs as a result of medications (pyridium) or foods (rhubarb, food coloring); blood in urine causes darkness; purulent matter makes it cloudy.

Odor

- May indicate certain foods (asparagus); old urine smells like ammonia. Diabetic and ketotic urine has a sweet odor.

pH

■ pH is normally around 6 and is slightly acidic.

CLINICAL NURSING IMPLICATIONS

■ Vegetarian diets may give a higher pH. Bacteria found in urinary tract infections creates alkaline urine, except *Escherichia coli*.

Blood

■ Normally not present in urine.

CLINICAL NURSING IMPLICATIONS

■ May indicate trauma in the urinary tract system. It is important to rule out contamination by menstrual fluid in females. This test is used with clients on heparin, warfarin sodium, or to note active bleeding in those with bleeding disorders.

Protein

■ Normally not present in urine.

CLINICAL NURSING IMPLICATIONS

■ Protein in urine may indicate renal disease. This test is used during prenatal visits to screen for toxemia.

Glucose

■ Normally not present in urine.

CLINICAL NURSING IMPLICATIONS

■ Results may be obtained via tablet, tape, or dipstick. Many drugs can interfere with this test, including aspirin, and many antibiotics.

Ketones

■ Normally not present in urine.

CLINICAL NURSING IMPLICATIONS

■ May indicate diabetic ketoacidosis. Some medications can give a false positive.

Urine Collection

Midstream

■ Begin by washing hands; always wear gloves.
■ Use three cotton balls covered with antiseptic solution.
■ For females, clean the meatal sides first, then directly over the urethra.
■ For males (if uncircumcised, retract foreskin), clean from the urethral opening away from the orifice with three cotton balls.
■ Give client a sterile container to void in.

POINT TO PONDER

Drugs with names ending in -mycin often give elevated urinary glucose levels. Blood testing for sugar is preferable because of its accuracy.

- Instruct the client to begin voiding and stop stream after 50 to 100 mL has been voided, and then void into a sterile collection container (30 mL). Have the client finish the remainder of void in toilet, commode, or urinal.

From Catheter

- Straight catheterization:
  Follow aseptic procedure (see Catheter section) and drain the urine into a sterile collection container.
- Indwelling catheter:
  Clamp tubing distal to collection port for several minutes only.
  Clean the collection port with an alcohol or iodine prep.
  Aspirate urine pooled in the area of the collection port with a sterile syringe and inject urine into specimen collection sterile container.

💡 **POINT TO PONDER**

Make sure sample is refrigerated after collection if it is not sent to the laboratory immediately.

▶ SAFETY TIP

Don't clamp catheter for longer than several minutes.

Catheters

Foley Catheter (indwelling and straight catheter)

- Begin client teaching before catheterizing and instruct client about the procedure and ways to relax. Teach deep breathing during procedure to decrease resistance.
- Assemble equipment.
- Position client comfortably, providing for adequate privacy.
- Place tray between legs and open equipment, including catheter.
- Lubricate the catheter.
- Clean the meatus.
- Insert the catheter until urine flows. Remove catheter when urine stops flowing if the order is for straight catheterization.
- Inflate balloon with sterile water only if indwelling Foley catheter is ordered.
- Attach to a drainage collection bag, and hang the bag below the level of the bladder.

▶ SAFETY TIP

Always keep the collection bag below the bladder level at all times to prevent the backward flow of urine into the bladder.

- Provide catheter care every shift, including cleansing the meatus around the catheter and removing any drainage or crusting.

X-ray of the Abdomen

- Flat plate of abdomen, or kidney, ureters, and bladder.
- (KUB) x-ray. This x-ray may be called a scout film and is used to visualize anatomic structures.

Excretory Urogram, Intravenous Pyelogram (IVP)

- This procedure is performed to evaluate the kidney structure.
- Clients should be assessed for allergy to iodine and shellfish; be kept NPO for 8 hours; and have a bowel evacuation as ordered.

Management post-procedure

- Encourage high-volume PO intake or increase IV fluids to clear dye quickly to decrease the possibility of renal reaction/failure (especially important in the elderly). Check vital signs regularly.

Cystoscopy and Urethroscopy

- Performed to view the urinary tract and to remove obstructions.
- Postprocedure management:
  Observe and report bleeding (pink tinge is expected, but clots or blood is abnormal).
  If a urinary tract infection occurs after the procedure, it will usually occur in 48 to 72 hours. Assess for typical complaints, an elevated temperature, shaking, and chills.

Renal Biopsy

- Procedure performed to obtain specimens for pathology.
- Postprocedure care includes keeping the client on bedrest for 8 hours and ensuring that he or she lies still for at least 4 hours.

Hemodialysis

- This process will help to remove waste products and excess fluid.
- An arteriovenous (AV) shunt/AV graft/AV fistula or subclavian catheter may be used to provide access to the bloodstream. AV shunts/grafts/fistulas are usually placed in the arm.

POINT TO PONDER

Proper position is supine with a sandbag or additional padding over site, or lying on the side on which the procedure was performed to minimize postprocedure bleeding.

▶ SAFETY TIP

Do not obtain blood pressures in arm with graft/fistula.

Client complaints of weakness, lightheadedness, and hyper- or hypotension indicate dialysis disequilibrium syndrome.

- Management for dialysis:
  Monitor vital signs both pre- and postprocedurally, obtain weights, and report and record information.
  Check sites after the procedure for hematomas or bleeding, and report immediately if noted.

▶ SAFETY TIP

Emergency equipment at the bedside includes a bulldog clamp in case an AV shunt becomes dislodged.

Peritoneal Dialysis

- The physician inserts a tube/catheter approximately 2 inches below the navel, and a warm dialysate is introduced into the abdomen.
- Check client weight and vital signs pre- and postprocedurally.
- During infusion, observe and report client complaints of cramping (solution is running in too fast), weakness (solution is too cold), or no return (peritoneal catheter may be blocked).

Urinary Disorders ▶

Urinary Tract Infection (Cystitis)

Data Collection

- Assess for pain, urgency, frequency, and burning with urination.
- Urine will be cloudy and foul smelling.
- Urinalysis may reveal occult blood and bacteria in sample.
- Nursing management includes teaching women to wipe from front to back with toilet tissue (least to most contaminated area).
- Encourage fluid intake to 3 liters per day unless contraindicated.
- Preventive measures may also include:
  Proper clothing: wear cotton-padded underwear.
  No bubble baths.
  Empty bladder after sex and do not delay voiding when urge occurs.

POINTS TO PONDER

The elderly often present with confusion as the first sign of UTI.

In pregnancy, dilation of the ureter and kidney will predispose the person to UTI.

Nephrolithiasis

- Stones that develop in the kidney may lodge within the ureters or the kidneys themselves.

Data Collection

- Client complaints may include flank pain and chills.
- Urine may contain frank blood (hematuria).

Management

- Encourage the client to ambulate to help move stone down ureter.
- Stones can be removed by ureteral catheter basket via cystoscopy.
- Extracorporeal shock wave lithotripsy smashes stones.

Acute Renal Failure

Oliguric Stage (low-output phase)

- This stage occurs when kidneys fail to produce urine.

Data Collection

- Client may complain of nausea and vomiting, confusion, or headache.
- Weight gain (may indicate sodium and fluid retention).
- Irregular pulse could indicate excess potassium in bloodstream.
- A complaint of warmness and burning in extremities may indicate magnesium excess.
- Note decreasing urinary output (oliguria) and signs of CHF.

Diuretic Stage (high-output phase)

- This stage begins when urine output is greater than 500 mL in one day.

Data Collection

- Output may go as high as 5 liters or more per day.
- Watch for a severely dehydrated appearance.
- Client will be rehydrated with intravenous fluids. Maintain a strict intake and output, and assist in keeping intake above output amounts.

Recovery Stage

- Final stage of reversible renal failure, lasts several months to years. Monitor and note changes as they occur.

Chronic Renal Failure

Management

- Prevent infections by maintaining good client hygiene and skin care (bathe in warm water with or without bath oil (no soap) to decrease itchiness per order.
- Perform invasive tasks using aseptic techniques.
- Assist with preparing dialysis (hemo- and peritoneal dialysis).
- Assist in maintaining fluid and sodium restriction.
- Observe and report signs and symptoms of metabolic acidosis, confusion, or other changes in mental status.

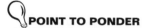

POINT TO PONDER

Report any changes immediately.

POINT TO PONDER

Report any changes immediately.

POINT TO PONDER

Many of the problems seen in chronic renal failure are the same as those in the oliguric stage of acute renal failure but are more severe and will not resolve without dialysis.

POINTS TO PONDER

Clients who are not able to void should never receive any supplemental potassium.

NO "P" MEANS NO "K."

Do not administer a Fleet enema as it contains sodium.

Anatomy, Physiology, Pathophysiology ▶ **Eyes**

Eyeball	The internal portion (back of the eye); includes the retina, optic disc, optic nerve, and fluid.
Sclera	The white of the eye.
Iris	The colored part of the eye.
Cornea	The transparent membrane covering the lens.
Lens	The biconvex structure that provides for focusing and directing light into the back of the eye.

Disorders/ Variations

Eyeballs	Will appear sunken in dehydrated client.
Lids	May appear to cover eyeballs in hypothyroidism.
	Yellow plaques are associated with hyperlipidemia or normal aging process.
Lacrimal gland	Decreased secretions in aging (dry eye syndrome) managed with "natural tears" drops.
Conjunctiva	Pale: anemia.
	Yellow: liver disease, jaundice.
	Red: infection/conjunctivitis.
	Bloody: subconjunctival hemorrhage.
Cornea	Grayish discolorations around edge are associated with arcus senilis (normal aging changes).
Lens	Decreased ability to focus on objects.
	Nearsightedness (myopia): able to see near objects but not able to see far objects.
	Farsightedness (hyperopia): able to see far objects but not able to see near objects.
Sclera	Normally whitish, but blue color may be seen in newborns and young children (thin sclera).

Ears

External ear	Portion of the ear that receives sound.
Middle ear	Contains the tympanic membrane, ossicles, eustachian tube, and mastoid bone.
Inner ear	Contains the cochlea, labyrinth, fluids, and the auditory nerve pathway.

Disorders/Variations

External ear	Otitis externa or swimmer's ear.
Middle ear	Otitis media, mastoiditis, and perforated eardrums.
Inner ear	Presbycusis (loss of high-frequency sounds), ototoxicity, and old-age hearing loss.

Data Collection, Procedures, and Treatments ▶ **Eyes**

Data Collection

■ Vision screening is recommended at least once per year in children and every other year in adults.

- Subjective: assess for complaints such as blurring of vision, blind spots, halo rings, headaches. Note use of glasses, last eye exam, history of glaucoma, injury, or cataracts.
- Objective: visual acuity is tested using a Snellen chart (20/20 normal).

Pupils

- Measure for size and reaction to light.
- Sluggish pupils associated with neurologic disorders and alcohol or drug abuse.
- Pupils will not react to light in some blindness, dense (discolored lens) cataracts, or severe neurologic dysfunction.
- Check pupils for reaction with flashlight. Normally, they will constrict with light.

Applying Eye Patches

- Wash hands thoroughly.
- Assemble supplies and equipment and put on gloves.
- Explain the procedure and indication for it.
- Have client close eye, then apply pad.
- Apply tape from middle of forehead to outer cheek.

Instilling Eye Drops

- Check order carefully.
- Abbreviations: OD, right eye; OS, left eye; OU, both eyes.
- Check medication carefully for proper strength.
- Wash hands and put on gloves.
- Have the client tilt head back to receive drops.
- Hold tissue in dominant hand below eye to catch additional drops and pull lower lid out.
- Brace the hand performing the instillation against client's cheek or forehead to minimize errors and contamination of eye medication.
- Maintain sterility of eye medication, drops, or ointments.
- Instill eye drops into area of conjunctival sac.
- When applying ointment, apply to lower lid in ribbon-like fashion.
- After application, have client keep eye closed for 3 minutes to prevent medication from being pushed into lacrimal duct collection area.
- Discard gloves, wash hands, and document administration.

Ears

Data Collection

- Subjective: assess for complaints of hearing loss, ringing of ears (tinnitis), discharge, ear pain, nausea and vomiting, and vertigo.
- Objective: acuity (hearing) is assessed using whispered voice, spoken voice, and watch tick.

POINTS TO PONDER

Totally blind means unable to see at all.

Legally blind means not able to see better than 20/200 with corrected vision.

POINT TO PONDER

Instill drops before instilling ointments; when applying more than one eye medication, wait at least 5 minutes between drops and 15 minutes between ointments.

Instilling Eardrops

- Assemble equipment.
- Make sure solution is at room temperature.
- Explain the procedure.
- Place client in a side-lying position.
- Hold the dropper 1 cm above ear.
- Pull the auricle upward and backward (in adults).
- Instill the drops and apply pressure to the tragus for 3 to 5 minutes.
- Wipe all excess drops away from ear.
- Contraindication for instilling drops is a known or suspected rupture of the tympanic membrane.

Heent and Special Senses Disorders ▶

Eye Disorders

Conjunctivitis	"Red eye" or "pink eye" seen in acute infections.
Cataracts	Opacity or clouding of the lens that is seen in older adults which gradually impairs vision.
Strabismus	Eye deviations seen in children with muscle weaknesses (lazy eye).
Nystagmus	Involuntary rapid movements of the eyeball.

Cataracts

- Data collection should assess for blurred vision, reading difficulties, and night blindness.

▶ SAFETY TIP

Identify self when entering room.

Keep room dimly lit and keep client oriented.

Keep call bell within easy reach.

- Maintain eye patch per order postoperatively.

Glaucoma

- This disorder is caused by an increase in the pressure within the eyeball itself and will cause blindness if not treated with medications.
- Administer all eye medications as ordered.
- Closed-angle glaucoma is a medical emergency; refer to an ophthalmologist/emergency department immediately.

Ear Disorders

Hearing Loss

- Communicating with client:
    Get client's attention at beginning of communication.

Face the client directly.

Speak slowly and articulate words.

Keep volume down and pitch down (high-frequency losses are most common).

Skull

◀ **Anatomy, Physiology, and Pathophysiology**

- Provides protection of contents from direct injury and is a closed cavity that leaves little room for swelling in times of injury, resulting in increased intracranial pressure (IICP).

Blood Supply

- Supplied by four major arteries: the carotid arteries in the neck and the vertebral arteries in the spinal column.

Brain and Brain Stem Structures

Frontal lobe	Judgment, emotions, and some motor function, including a speech center.
Parietal lobe	Sensory and speech areas.
Temporal lobe	Long-term memory and intellect, and understanding speech of others.
Occipital lobe	Area that receives visual stimuli.
Midbrain	Some cranial nerves begin in this area.
Medulla oblongata	Center of cardiac, respiratory, vasomotor, and automatic responses.
Pons	Regulates respiration (inspiration and expiration depth).
Hypothalamus	Maintains internal environment control and behavior.
Hypophysis pituitary	Controls growth and lactation.

Cerebral Spinal Fluid

- Normally clear in color, specific gravity of 1.003 to 1.008; contains protein, glucose, chlorides.
- Should not have white or red blood cells.

Walking Abnormalities

Type/name	Examples of Cause	Description
Hemiplegia gait	Cerebral vascular accident	Arm rigid (spastic paralysis) and leg on same side not easily lifted
Propulsive gait	Parkinson's disease	Movements as if person is going to fall forward

Tremors

- Intention tremor: tremors appear in multiple sclerosis.
- Resting tremor: tremors occur in Parkinson's disease clients and in clients suffering side effects from psychotropic medications.

Neurologic Signs

◀ **Data Collection, Procedures, and Treatments**

- Pupils usually react to light equally and quickly in both eyes. Abnormalities can include a "fixed" or nonreactive pupil occurring in blindness and with brain damage; unequal pupils that often indicates increased intracranial pressure (IICP); and pinpoint pupils, which are observed in clients being treated for glaucoma.

Glasgow Coma Scale

- Scale used to assess the level of consciousness in persons who may be going into, are in, or are coming out of a coma.

Computerized Tomography (CT Scan)

- CT scan is used to visualize intracranial bleeding masses and herniation of the brain. **If a dye is used, ask about allergy to iodine/shellfish.** This procedure is somewhat noisy and the client can feel closed in. Claustrophobia is a contraindication.

Electroencephalogram (EEG)

- Used to evaluate brain activity and to rule out seizure disorders. Can be done awake or asleep. Numerous leads with gel on adhesive patches are attached to various areas of the head, after which a head wrap is applied. Keep client still during test. Used to assess for seizure disorders.

Magnetic Resonance Image (MRI)

- Most accurate method of evaluating structures of the brain, brain stem, and spinal cord. **Contraindicated in clients with metal objects such as pins, rods, hip prostheses, and in those with electrical appliances such as pacemakers.** Noisy procedure with problems similar to those seen in the CT scan.

Lumbar Puncture

- This procedure is performed to obtain a cerebral spinal fluid specimen. Obtained by a physician. Postprocedurally, client lies flat for 4 to 6 hours (logrolling for turning is permitted). If headache occurs, continue bedrest for up to 24 hours or as ordered.

Blood Tests

Phenytoin (Dilantin) Level

- Normal: 10 to 20 µg/mL for therapeutic effect.

CLINICAL NURSING IMPLICATIONS

- Note signs and symptoms of toxicity, including slurred speech, nausea, nystagmus, ataxia, confusion, and dizziness. Should be monitored routinely once maintained.

Neurologic Disorders ▶ ### Seizure Disorder

Tonic–Clonic (Grand Mal)

DATA COLLECTION

- May be preceded by an "aura" (premonition) such as visual, auditory, or tactile hallucinations. Seizure begins with a cry or a fall to the floor. Breathing pattern changes; client may lose bowel and bladder control. Lasts several minutes (usually 2 or less), and confusion after a seizure is likely.

Absence (Petit Mal)

DATA COLLECTION

- Usually begins around ages 4 to 12 and results in a sudden appearance of "day dreaming" or staring blankly off into space (which is the seizure activity).

▶ SAFETY TIP

Think of keeping the airway open as the major priority.

MANAGEMENT

- Have an airway available.
- Protect from injury by moving furniture.
- Loosen shirt or blouse collar and tie.
- Turn client on side or turn head to side for protection from injury and aspiration.
- Look for Medic-Alert bracelet.
- Provide a calm environment when consciousness returns.
- Call for help and an ambulance if seizure doesn't stop after 5 minutes in pregnant clients or diabetics.
- Expect postseizure confusion; reorient client.
- Seizure precautions include padded side rails for bed, which should be raised during seizure activity.

GENERAL CONSIDERATIONS FOR ANY SEIZURE DISORDER

- Teach client to avoid swimming in deep water; to take showers rather than baths (but do not shower when alone); to restrict driving to seizure-free periods (determined by state of license); not to operate machinery; if smoker, not to smoke alone; and not to ingest alcohol.
- Medical management of seizures involves medications (Dilantin, phenobarbital, and other antiseizure medications).

Cerebral Vascular Accident (CVA)

- Risk factors are associated with hypertension, hypotension, and other vascular diseases.

Data Collection

SUBJECTIVE AND OBJECTIVE FINDINGS

- **Early:** headache, facial droop, transient loss of voluntary muscles, transient ischemic attacks (TIAs).

💡 **POINT TO PONDER**

Do not force anything into the mouth, give liquids, or attempt to hold the tongue.

- **Late:** Loss of consciousness, hemiplegia, aphasia, seizures, nuchal rigidity (neck stiffness indicates meningeal irritation).

Management

- Provide a good oxygen supply to the brain by maintaining airway, breathing, and circulation and providing supplemental oxygen as ordered.
- Initially, monitor vital signs and neurologic signs every 2 hours or more frequently.

Right-sided CVA

- Right-sided brain damage with left-sided problems.
- Physical problems include left-sided neglect (clients forget that they have lost the use of their left side). Some form of restraint is frequently ordered (seat belts in wheel chairs, side rails on bed, bedside tables in front of chairs).
- Emotional changes lead to frequent crying. Inform family that this is due to neurologic damage and not necessarily due to depression.
- Left-sided hemianopsia (loss of half the visual field):
  Client will not see objects in the normal visual field unless they are on the right side. Place meal items, utensils, pens, and paper on the right side so they can be seen. Approach the client from the unaffected side (right). Place the client in bed so that the unaffected side (ie, right side) is closest to the door and client can see people come and go.
- Left hemiplegia or hemiparesis:
  Loss of function on the left side of body. Clients need assistance with ADLs, ambulation, and transfers. Be alert to impulsive behavior, and avoid injury with mild restraints, *if prescribed*. Clients will develop left arm edema if arm is not properly suspended or held in lap.

▶ SAFETY TIP

Right CVA clients are a safety risk because they may deny the extent of their problems (left-sided neglect).

Left-sided CVA

- Left-sided brain damage with right-sided problems.
- Major problem associated with left CVA is a communication deficit.
- Aphasia (loss of speech):
  Client may present with difficulty understanding words, being able to express words, or both; may not be able to understand directions. Speak slowly and look directly at the client to get his or her attention. Expect frustration and swearing. Alert family to angry outbursts and frustration. Keep questions short.

- Depression/anger:

  Client may become depressed because of an awareness that something is wrong. Antidepressants are sometimes used. Crying is usually a result of depression and fear. Client may be quick to anger and get easily frustrated.

- Overcautiousness:

  Client is aware of major problems associated with hemiplegia and may be fearful of injury. The client requires a great deal of encouragement. Use short, direct questions in the initial stages of communication.

- Right-sided hemianopsia (loss of half the visual field):

  Client will not see objects in the normal visual field unless they are on left side. Place meal items, utensils, pens, and paper on the left side so they can be seen. Approach the client from the left side. Place the client in bed so that the right side is closest to the door and client can see people come and go.

- Right-sided hemiplegia:

  Client is unable to ambulate without assistance. Nurse should stand on the left side and support the client when needed.

General Rules for Both Types of CVAs

- Place affected leg in slight internal rotation with knee flexed when in bed.
- Watch for hypotension and orthostatic changes when getting up.
- Keep transfer chair on unaffected (good) side so client can utilize the undamaged leg and arm.
- A cane is held on the undamaged side and advanced at the same time as the affected leg is moved forward.
- Braces are placed on leg (shin splints too) to provide rigid stability and to prevent foot drop.

Increased Intracranial Pressure (IICP)

- Any condition causing swelling within the brain or obstruction of outflow of CSF.

Data Collection

- **Earliest:**

  Restlessness and agitation.
  Change in level of consciousness.

- **Middle:**

  Pupils react sluggishly/slowly to light reflex.
  Early morning headache.

- **Later:**

  Change in vital signs, including bradycardia, increased systolic pressure and widening pulse pressure, and decreased respirations.
  Diffuse headache and projectile vomiting.
  Visual disturbances.

Management

- Maintain airway and breathing:
  Head of bed elevated at 30 degrees (side-lying position OK).
  Don't position the neck in flexion.
  Have oxygen and suction available at bedside.
  Fluid restriction of 1500 mL per day or less is usually ordered.
- Monitor mental status:
  Neurologic exam and vital signs every 15 minutes.
  Glasgow Coma Scale assessments may be ordered.
  Notify physician of significant changes.

Closed Head Injury

- Head trauma results in changes in personality and difficulty with mentation and memory.

Data Collection

- **Epidural hematoma** signs and symptoms:
  Client becomes lethargic or lapses into unconsciousness within hours and up to several days after trauma.
- **Subdural hematoma** signs and symptoms:
  Client becomes lethargic or lapses into unconsciousness within several days to months after trauma.

Spinal Cord Injury/Transection

- In transection, the nerve pathways are totally severed at a specific level.
- Injury level impairments and managment:
  Quadriplegia: potential for respiratory arrest, no (or minimal) hand movement preserved; usually requires total assistance, electric wheelchair, and bowel and bladder managment.
  Paraplegia: client will have the capacity to self-propel a wheelchair, perform ADLs, transfer self from bed to chair, and breathe normally; can be totally independent.

Guillain–Barré Syndrome

- A weakness and paralysis that begins in the lower legs and moves up the body to the head; usually occurs soon after a viral infection.
- May cause respiratory dysfunction/arrest.
- Maintain proper alignment and postioning to prevent contractures, prevent skin problems, and manage bowel and bladder incontinence.

MUSCULOSKELETAL SYSTEM

Anatomy, Physiology, ▶ and Pathophysiology

Muscles

- Three types: *skeletal* (voluntary) muscles, such as the arms and legs; *smooth* (involuntary) muscles, such as in the GI tract; and *cardiac* (involuntary) muscles, such as the heart.

Selected Muscle Disorders

Contractures	The muscle fibers or connective tissue become shortened and will cause pain when the client tries to stretch or exercise the muscle.
Atrophy	The muscle gets smaller and weaker.
Spasticity	The muscle overcontracts; occurs with some neurologic or nerve disorders.
Dystrophy	The muscle becomes weak and lacks coordination.

Bone disorders

Fractures	Breaks in the bone, named by type.
Osteoporosis	In the aging process, especially in women who lack estrogen, the bone (matrix) becomes thinner and can fracture easier.
Osteomyelitis	Infection of bone.

Joint Disorders

Arthritis	Inflammation or pain in the joints; can be diagnosed as osteoarthritis, rheumatoid arthritis, or septic arthritis.
Sprain	Rupture of the ligaments in and around the area of joints.

Assessing CSMs (Neurovascular Checks)

◄ **Data Collection, Procedures, and Treatments**

Circulation	Check for skin color, temperature, pulses, and edema.
Sensation	Evaluate the extremities (usually hands and feet) to determine the ability to sense touch.
Movement	Note the motion of an extremity and compare it with the opposite side.

Range of Motion

Type	Description
Abduction	Movement away from midline of body
Adduction	Movement toward midline of body
Supination	Palms upward
Pronation	Palms downward
Inversion	Turning foot inward
Eversion	Turning foot outward
External rotation	Moving and turning away from midline of body

X-rays

- Visualize bones and some soft tissues.

Bone Scan

- Picks up increased levels of radioisotopes in areas of cancer.

Electromyography

- Measures muscle response to electrical stimulus.

Casts and Care

- When clients suffer a bone fracture, have an amputation, or suffer from some types of muscle injuries, they are often placed in a cast. Casting immobilizes extremities, muscles, and bones and allows them to heal.

Types of Casts	Use
Long: arm or leg	Long bone fractures
Short: arm or leg	Wrist fractures, foot fractures, ankle fractures
Hinged cast	Corrects contractures of knee by setting hinge setting and gradually changing setting to improve stretch
Spica (involves the trunk of the body)	Immobilizes the pelvic area including the hip after surgery; used more often in children than adults
Body cast	Used to immobilize spine after trauma or surgery

- Types of casts:
  Synthetic casts set/dry within 15 minutes; weight bearing is allowed in 30 minutes.
  Plaster casts set within 15 minutes; drying time is up to 72 hours (no weight bearing allowed until then).
- Cast should dry and set in air only; don't use hairdryers, sunlamps, or other outside sources of heat.
  "Petaling" of the cast edge is done only after the cast is completely dry and is used to prevent abrasions from forming at the edges of cast openings. Overlapping tape strips are applied at the top of the opening of the cast resembling the petals of a flower.
- Evaluate for any complications that can occur with casting, such as infection (detected by feeling a warm area on cast, observing drainage on cast, or noting a foul-smelling odor from the cast); pain, paralysis, or paresthesia (tingling and numbness), which occurs in nerve damage; swelling (edema) near the top, bottom, or beyond the cast; and skin breakdown around the cast area.
- Specific care tips:
  Reposition the client every 2 hours during the setting/drying process and keep the cast open to air (do not cover).
  Maintain an elevated position for the cast during the first 24 to 72 hours to prevent edema; use of pillows or slings is appropriate (as ordered).
  Keep cast dry, and provide skin care every 4 hours.

POINT TO PONDER

Apply alcohol to skin areas around the edge of the cast (or under cast if bivalved). No lotions, creams, or oils as these soften skin and may increase breakdowns.

▶ SAFETY TIP

Handle cast with the flats or palms of hands. NO fingertips!

- Do not put anything in cast for pruritis/itching; use cool air dryers only.
- Push fluids to 3 liters per day unless contraindicated.
- Usual diet will be high protein, high carbohydrate.

- Make sure to keep cast dry with water-resistant materials such as plastic wraps; for infants, use double diapers or sanitary pads to absorb urine.
- Use fracture pans; position clients comfortably and pad the pan for additional comfort for those on bedrest.
- For catheterized clients, keep perineal area clean and dry and maintain strict intake and output measurements.

Crutch and Cane Walking

Gait/Activity	Procedure
For crutches:	
Two-point gait	Move right foot and left crutch forward at the same time, then move left foot and right crutch forward at the same time; start over again.
Three-point gait	Move affected foot (leg) and both crutches forward at the same time, then move unaffected leg forward; start over again.
Four-point gait	Move right crutch forward first, then left foot, then left crutch, then right foot; start over again.
Swing-to gait	Move right crutch first, then left crutch, then swing both legs up to crutches at the same time; start over again.
Swing-through gait	Move right crutch first, then left crutch, then swing both legs through crutches (past crutches) to end ahead of them; start over again.
Stair climbing	Going up stairs: proceed with unaffected (good) leg first, then advance crutches and affected (bad) leg after.
Going down stairs	Proceed with both crutches and affected (bad) leg first, then advance unaffected (good) leg.

Using a Cane

- Hold the cane on unaffected (good) side. Move the cane and affected (bad) leg at the same time first (simultaneously), then advance the good leg.
- The cane handle should be held with the elbow flexed at 30 degrees; it should be at the level of the femur.

Using a Walker

- The top of the walker should be at the same level as the cane (head at femur level) with the elbow flexed at 30 degrees.

Traction

- The two types of traction are skin traction, in which the weights are attached to belts, pads, and pulleys; and skeletal traction, in which surgery places pins, rods, and wires that come out of the body, to which the ropes are attached.

► SAFETY TIPS

Weights must hang freely (keep them off the ground). If they are on the floor, move the client up in bed away from the weight to move it off the floor.

Never release weights unless ordered (maintain traction).

POINT TO PONDER

Two-point gait is used for a bilateral amputee with a prosthesis.

POINT TO PONDER

Three-point gait is used for a non-weight–bearing person with a fracture of the leg or hip.

POINT TO PONDER

Four-point gait is used for patients with polio and cerebral palsy.

POINT TO PONDER

Swing-to gait is used by the paraplegic with leg braces.

POINT TO PONDER

Swing-through gait is used by the paraplegic with leg braces.

POINT TO PONDER

Remember: THE GOOD GO TO HEAVEN (move good leg first when going up); THE BAD GO TO HELL (move crutches and bad leg first going down).

POINT TO PONDER

When using a walker, advance it 6 to 12 inches and then move into it.

Common Types of Traction	Use
Buck's traction	Fractured femur or hip
Bryant's traction	Used with infants and small children and is similar to Buck's; elevates both lower extremities in a 90-degree fashion (make sure buttocks touch the bed by being able to slide hand between buttocks and bed)
Russell's traction	Fractured femurs, tibias; knee or hip immobilization
Pelvic traction	Lower back pain and strain
Halo traction	Used to immobilize spinal cord and column

Assess for Complications of Traction

- Check for CSM; assess for deep vein thrombosis (calf tenderness) and infection around pin sites.

Orthopedic Disorders ▶ **Arthritis**

- Types include: rheumatoid, juvenile rheumatoid, and osteoarthritis.
- Rheumatoid arthritis stiffness occurs in the early morning and gets better during the day; the joints may swell and become very deformed. In osteoarthritis the stiffness gets worse as the day progresses and there is not as much swelling or deformity of joints.

Nursing Care Do's and Don'ts

- **Do** exercise joints with active range of motion.
- **Don't** exercise acutely inflamed joints (use proper positioning during the acute inflammatory episodes of rheumatoid arthritis).
- **Do** exercise regularly but not to the point that it becomes painful.
- **Do** exercise at a slow, steady pace.
- **Don't** exercise with weights unless ordered.
- **Do** a minimum of three or more joint ranges per day.

Fractures

Types	Description
Complete	The bone is completely separated
Greenstick	Looks like a green stick broken off the branch of a tree
Comminuted	The bone is broken into fragments
Spiral	May be seen in children; related to abuse
Closed	No bone is protruding
Open	Bone is exposed
Compound	Skin has been broken (open fracture)
Compression	Bone collapses on itself (vertebrae)

POINT TO PONDER

Assess for the 5 Ps of fractures:
- Pain
- Pulse
- Pallor
- Parasthesia
- Paralysis

- Assess for the following complications after a fracture:

Hemorrhage	Assess for shock, evaluate vital signs, and observe for signs of bleeding
Pulmonary embolism	Assess for shortness of breath, anxiety, and restlessness
Infection	Assess for foul-smelling drainage and discharge in areas of skin breaks

Hip Replacement

- Postoperative positioning:
    Use only an elevated toilet seat, and use footstools to keep hip in less than 90-degree flexion or chair which can recline while lifting feet, and avoid low chairs.
    Keep client off the operated side unless ordered.
    Don't elevate head of bed and foot of bed at same time.
    Remind client to not cross legs or bend forward.

► SAFETY TIP

Always keep the hip in abducted position (must avoid adduction, internal rotation, and flexion).

Amputation of Lower Extremities

- Types: Above the knee (AKA) and below the knee (BKA)
- Postoperative care:
    Monitor vital signs every 15 minutes until stable, then every 2 hours for first 24 hours, then every 4 hours.
    Keep the stump elevated for first 24 hours; do not elevate stump with pillows after first 24 hours.
- To prevent contractures:
    Client can be placed prone (face down) for 15 minutes, four times per day if able to tolerate (especially AKA).
    Clients should be encouraged to do active ROM of extremity.

POINTS TO PONDER

Notify supervisor for complaints of pain. Any pain lasting longer than 2 days should be evaluated for infection.

Phantom pain is real to the clients.

SAFETY TIP

Monitor for bleeding and report immediately.

Apply pressure directly over the area of bleeding.

Notify charge nurse or physician ASAP.

Keep a tourniquet at the bedside for bleeding.

- Stump of extremity is wrapped to shape the stump so it will fit into a prosthesis appropriately. Use an Ace bandage (elastic wrap) 4 to 6 inches wide.
- Help clients adjust to body image by encouraging them to talk about, look at, and touch amputated area when ready.

Immunologic System

Anatomy, Physiology, ▶
and Pathophysiology

- The immunologic system is organized to create a resistance against infections and invasions of foreign organisms or agents.
- T cells and B cells are lymphocytes that respond to inflammation and infection.
- Involves the antigen (foreign agent)–antibody (body response to invasion) reaction.

Data Collection, Procedures, ▶
and Treatments

- Enzyme-linked immunosorbent assay (ELISA) is used to find the antibodies causing human immunodeficiency virus (HIV).
    Positive HIV test doesn't indicate whether the person has the disease or is only infected with the virus.
- Erythrocyte sedimentation rate (ESR) determines inflammatory states of all causes.
- Skin tests such as a tuberculin test determine whether antibodies exist for specific infections.

Allergic and Anaphylactic Responses

- Subjective:
    Itchiness (pruritis); stuffiness; runny nose; cough; difficulty breathing; history of allergies to foods, pollens, medications, and environmental agents.
- Objective:
    Skin rashes, hives, nasal discharges, infections, inflammation, and respiratory findings such as wheezing and dyspnea.
- Always determine and identify those with history of allergies (including food and drugs), family history of allergies, or history of environmental exposure creating reactions.

▶ SAFETY TIP

Prevention: Special identification bands such as Medic-Alert bracelets; tag chart for those with allergies.

Note drugs that client has had allergy to and cross-index similar drugs.

Management for Reactions

- Notify physician.
- Check vital signs.
- Administer oxygen per order of physician.
- **Have the following available:**
    Epinephrine (per order).
    Benadryl (per order).

Acquired Immunodeficiency Syndrome (AIDS)

- High-risk categories: homosexuals, bisexuals, IV drug users, individuals who received blood transfusions prior to 1985, hemophiliacs, and newborns of mothers who are HIV positive.

Complaints and Findings

- Early complaints: none; HIV-positive blood test.
- Complaints/findings with disease include fungal/candidal infections (thrush or repeated vaginal infections), pneumonia (PCP), tuberculosis, fatigue, weight loss, unexplained bruising (Kaposi's sarcoma).

Diagnostic Tests

- Low WBC count—usually less than 1500/mm^3.
- T4 cell count less than 300 mm^3.
- T4/T8 cell ratio less than 1.
- Positive ELISA test.

Management

- Nutrition: improve appetite by offering small, frequent meals. Avoid hot/cold foods, spicy foods, and perform mouth care for those with thrush.
- Respiratory infections/PCP: avoid large crowds and administer medications as ordered. Encourage compliance to medical treatment plan. Observe for difficulty breathing and nonproductive cough.
- Fungal/candidal infections: good mouth care, swish and swallow antifungals, provide tepid liquids, avoid acidic foods; may require NG tube in severe disorder.
- Diarrhea: encourage fluids, monitor episodes of diarrhea, and report.

Medications

- Zidovudine (AZT, Retrovir) decreases amount of HIV in system and slows progression of disease.
- Amphotericin B as an antifungal.
- Trimethoprim/sulfamethoxazole (Bactrim, Septra) used to treat pneumocystis infections.
- Interferon and interleukin-2 are used to bring remission to disease.
- Isoniazid (INH) for prophylactic use when client is at risk for TB infection.
- Provide emotional support and client teaching of above and ways to prevent transmission.

POINTS TO PONDER

Health care professionals maintain universal precautions.

Teach all ages to wear condoms and avoid high-risk sex acts.

Avoid use of IV drugs (illicit) and never share needles.

Anatomy, Physiology, and ▶ Pathophysiology

Skin Components and Layers

Epidermis	Outer layer of skin protects from environmental threats.
Dermis	Layer of highly vascular tissue supplying nourishment to the dermis; has sensory fibers and motor fibers throughout.
Subcutaneous	Fatty-like layer of tissue that provides for keeping heat in and protection against trauma.
Appendages	Sweat glands, sebaceous glands, hair, and nails.

Types and Description of Selected Primary Lesions

- Macules: flat, nonraised, less than 1 cm.
    Examples: measles, freckles.

- Papules: raised, less than 1 cm.
    Examples: warts, moles.

- Vesicles: small, fluid-filled blisters.
    Examples: herpes blisters, chickenpox.

- Nodules: extend deeper into skin, hard, greater than 0.5 cm but less than 2 cm.
    Example: small nodules on finger joints observed in some arthritic conditions.

- Cysts: fluid- or exudate-filled sacs.
    Example: sebaceous cyst.

- Pustule: elevated, pus-filled.
    Example: acne.

- Tumor: elevated, larger than 2 cm.
    Examples: carcinoma, lipoma.

Description of Selected Skin Abnormalities/Variations

Alopecia	Hair loss/baldness.
Carbuncle	A cluster of boils (furuncles).
Cellulitis	Infection of skin tissue.
Hirsutism	Excessive hair growth in women.
Hyperkeratosis	Hypertrophy of skin.
Keloids	Hypertrophy of scar tissue.
Stria	Elevated or depressed lines in skin (stretch marks).
Vitiligo	Areas of nonpigmentation.

Abnormal Skin Colors

Cyanosis	*Central cyanosis* due to cardiac, respiratory, or hematologic disorders. *Peripheral cyanosis* due to vascular disorders such as Raynaud's disease.
Jaundice	Related to elevated bilirubin levels as seen in newborns and in adults with liver or gallbladder disease.
Pallor	Related to loss of circulation, poor pigmentation, and hematologic disorders such as anemia.
Rubor	Red color often associated with inflammation.

Types and Descriptions of Wound Drainage

Type	Description	Example
Serous	Watery and clear	Clear discharge leaking from the skin of clients with low albumin, burns, or large open wounds
Sanguineous	Bloody	Ulcerations or wounds that have just occurred
Serosanguineous	Bloody drainage mixed with clear, making it appear thinner than sanguineous drainage	Wound in which the acute bleeding phase has ceased and early tissue repair is beginning
Purulent	Thick, nonbloody, protein rich	Wounds undergoing infection or inflammation

Subjective Data Collection

- Current complaint: onset, duration, location, severity, radiation or spread, pain, itch, burning sensation, redness, tingling, and numbness.

- Additional information: previous skin disorders, medication history, allergy history, family history of skin disorders, use of new products (soaps/detergents).

Objective Data Collection (inspection)

- Skin: color, temperature, moisture, turgor, lesions, scars, striae, lesions.

- Hair: amount, location, texture, color.

- Nails: shape, color, length, lesions, cleanliness of nail beds.

Wound Culture

- Swab of the wound drainage.

Clinical Nursing Implications

- The area around the wound is cleaned to prevent contamination; swab should be placed back in the tube to prevent contamination and spread of infection.

Biopsy

- Sample of living tissue to determine its type.

- Postbiopsy management:
  Check for bleeding around site.
  Assess and medicate for pain per order.
  Assess for evidence of infection at suture line or puncture site.

Skin Testing

- To determine allergies or responses to various antigens such as the tuberculin test.

- Two types of tests:
  The *patch test* will be read in 24 to 48 hours (used to detect allergy to substances).
  The *intradermal test* will be read in 48 to 72 hours (used to determine antigen response of a systemic nature).

- Instruct client to return at the appropriate time to have skin tests read. Positive reactions are usually red and raised or blistered.

Types of Dressings for Short- and Long-term Wound Care

Dry sterile dressing	A sterile dressing used to protect the wound from external contamination; usually applied after cleansing of the wound has been performed.
Transparent adhesive film dressing	A covering which prevents external contamination while allowing oxygen to enter.
Hydrocolloid dressing	Used to keep the wound moist and provide a barrier from outside.
Absorptive dressing	Used to absorb exudate and drainage while protecting the wound.
Wet-to-dry dressing	Used to draw exudate away from the wound surface and to dry area.

Therapeutic Baths

Type	Example	Use
Colloidal	Starch, baking soda	Relieves itching
Emollients	Alpha Keri	Relieves pruritis
		Moistens dry skin
Tar	Coal tar	Relieves pruritis; treats scales such as those of psoriasis

General Skin Care

- Hygiene: goal is to keep a clean, dry, intact skin surface; bathing with mild soaps can remove excess oil, dirt, bacteria, and odor.
- Bathing too frequently results in dryness and flaking.
- Drying areas after bathing, especially where skin meets skin, helps to prevent bacterial and fungal infections.
- Cut nails short to avoid damaging skin.
- Diet: well-balanced, especially with protein and vitamins (A, C, and B especially).
- Exposure: avoid overexposure to sun, chemicals, or other physical agents.

Integumentary Disorders ▶

Pruritic Conditions

- Itching usually associated with dryness, skin irritation, allergic reaction, or a deposit of chemical irritants on skin.

Management

- Wash with tepid water only (avoid soaps).
- Apply emollients and moisturizers to skin.
- Wear cotton clothing to allow for air circulation and for perspiration to dry.
- Employ cool soaks to inflamed areas for a cooling, soothing effect.
- Administer medications (with orders) to minimize itch (corticosteroids or antihistamines).

POINT TO PONDER

When making frequent dressing changes to an area, use Montgomery straps to eliminate the need for using tape with each dressing change.

POINT TO PONDER

Bathe clients with dry skin daily with water only, and apply emollients to moisturize skin.
Exception: Bathe older adults who have no other skin disorders with water only *every other day*, and apply emollients to moisturize skin.

Pressure Sores/Ulcers

Data Collection Information

- Prevention is the key.

- Assess for the following risk factors associated with development of ulcers/pressure sores in clients who actually (or potentially) have the following problems:
    Mental status changes
    Urinary incontinence
    Nutritional deficiencies
    Debility
    Age
    Numerous medical problems
    Exercise and activity intolerance

▶ SAFETY TIP

For the client on bedrest or restrictions, a major priority of care is to prevent pressure sore development.

Categories of Skin Breakdown and Pressure Sore Formation

Stage 1   Erythema development over bony prominence that blanches when pressure is applied.
Stage 2   Erythema over bony prominences that does not blanch when pressure is applied.
Stage 3   Ulceration stage in which skin is broken and blisters/bullae form (epidermis is affected).
Stage 4   Full-thickness ulcer formation has occurred, which extends beyond the epidermis and involves underlying structures as well.

- To prevent pressure sores:
    Get all clients out of bed as much as medical condition allows.
    Keep client off all bony prominences by creating and using a regular turning schedule (at least every 2 hours).
    Massage areas of pressure points at least once per shift to improve circulation to that area (unless there is evidence that a pressure sore is present).
    Avoid shearing forces (created by pulling and not lifting client) when moving in bed or wheelchair; this creates a breakdown of fragile blood vessels.
    Keep incontinent clients as dry as possible by checking every hour for dampness and changing damp clothing and linens.
    Apply emollients to prevent dryness of skin, and bathe client at least daily if incontinent of urine or stool.

Dermatitis

- *Contact dermatitis:* soaps, makeup, and poison ivy are examples.

- *Exfoliative dermatitis:* drug reactions and psoriasis are examples.

- *Stasis dermatitis:* venous conditions creating poor circulation is an example.

Burns

Types of Burns

- Thermal (flames, fire, steam, sun).
- Chemical (lye, chlorine, hydrochloric acid).
- Electrical (high-voltage lines, house current, home appliances).
- Radiation (nuclear reactor accidents, overexposure in areas of high radiation).

Depth of Burns

- First degree: superficial (sunburns).
- Second degree: dermal involvement (blisters forming after exposure to hot matches, touching stove).
- Third degree: muscle/bone/fascia involvement (prolonged exposure to heat/flames without relief, eg, gasoline explosions, major building fires).

► SAFETY TIP

If burn involves the neck or head, suspect inhalation injury.

Data Collection for Respiratory Involvement

- Observe for burns to upper chest, neck, or face; singed eyebrows, mustaches, facial hair, nasal hair; soot in sputum; hoarseness of speech; swelling of lips, mucosa, or throat; dyspnea; wheezing, stridor (crowing sound).

► SAFETY TIP

For clients suffering from inhalation burns, prepare for tracheostomy (have kit at bedside), administer oxygen, and transfer to burn trauma center ASAP.

- Rule of nines (to measure surface of burned area):

	%	Total
Entire head	9	9%
Torso (front)	18	18%
Torso (back)	18	18%
Arms (each)	9 (× 2)	18%
Legs (each)	18 (× 2)	36%
Perineum	1	1%
Total		100%

POINT TO PONDER

Parkland–Baxter method of fluid replacement for burn clients.

Calculated by multiplying the percent of body surface burned by weight of person (in kilograms) by 4 mL, which equals the amount of fluid to be delivered in 24 hours.

Example: A person weighing 60 kg burned on chest (18%), perineum (1%), both arms (front only) (4.5% times two = 9%), and entire head (9%), equals 37%.

Consequently: 37 × 60 × 4 mL = 8880 mL

8880 mL is the amount of fluid that must be delivered to this client in the first 24 hours to prevent a fluid volume deficit.

- Fluid replacement is critical to survival following burns.

Method of Fluid Delivery

- This intravenous fluid will be delivered in the following manner:

  1/2 of 24-hour total will be delivered in the first 8 hours (in above client, 4440 mL).

  1/4 of 24-hour total will be delivered in the second 8 hours (in above client, 2220 mL).

  1/4 of 24-hour total will be delivered in the third 8 hours (in above client, 2220 mL).

- When calculating the delivery of fluid, the 24-hour period begins at the time the burn occurred, not when the person is admitted to the hospital.

▶ SAFETY TIP

Initial intervention in burn situations: remove from the source of the burn. (Exception: do not attempt to pull a person away from high-tension wires. Shut off power if possible or call the electric company.)

Nursing Management Points

- Stop the burning process by covering the person or rolling him or her around on the ground.
- Check for airway, breathing, and circulation.
- Skin changes related to external radiation include redness, dryness, and complaints of warmth at the site of radiation are expected.

Managing External Radiation Client

▶ SAFETY TIP

Make sure to preserve all markings, do not wash off.

- Teach the client to wash the area with water only and to report feelings of warmth, burning, and difficulty swallowing to supervisor.
- Emollients may be applied per order (avoid powders, lotions, and creams), especially when the client complains of warmth and burning over an area.
- If radiation is around the neck or head, client may complain of dry mouth or difficulty swallowing. Instruct the client to use hard sugar candies and fluids and to avoid gravies, sauces, and irritating/astringent fluids such as lemon and glycerine solutions or alcohol-based products.

Psoriasis

- Silver and scaly lesions described as plaques (raised) appearing on the skin, which may involve the nails; usually occur on the scalp, elbows, knees, or sacrum.
- Managed using topical steroids, tars, and oatmeal baths or systemically with steroids or the antimetabolite drug methotrexate.

Nursing Management

- Avoid temperature extremes, encourage a well-balanced diet, prevent itching and scratching of lesions.
- Assist with body image disturbance related to unsightly scaling.
- Teach use of topical medications.
- Encourage client to stay in the sun as it discourages production of psoriasis scaling.
- Avoid use of combs for hair; use a soft-bristle brush to avoid damaging scales in scalp.

PART III

▶ Specialty Areas

- Psychosocial/Communication
- Elder Care Issues and Management Considerations
- Issues Related to Care of Children
- Reproduction and Maternity

This section is devoted to presentation of information in several specialty areas. The areas covered in Part III include material related to the pyschosocial and communication area, elder care, care of the child, and maternity considerations. Important information is presented in table format to assist in remembering the key points.

PSYCHOSOCIAL/COMMUNICATION

Erikson's Eight Stages of Psychosocial Development

Age	Developmental Tasks	Exhibited By
Birth to 1½ years	Trust versus mistrust	Trust: feeding with ease, able to sleep, overall happiness Mistrust: lack of weight gain, failure to thrive, poor eating, colic, poor sleep patterns
1½ to 3 years	Autonomy versus shame and doubt	Autonomy: self-control, need to perform activities for self, able to say "no," ritualistic behavior Shame and doubt: fear, insecurity, negative in beliefs, stubborn, many temper tantrums, low tolerance to frustration, overactive, impulsive
3 to 6 years	Initiative versus guilt	Initiative: gets along with others, begins learning rules, limited and short temper tantrums Guilt: anger, shame, anxiety, lack of initiative, nightmares, eating and elimination problems
6 to 12 years	Industry versus inferiority	Industry: self-confident, pride in accomplishing tasks, self-control, cooperative, attention seeking, competent in play Inferiority: moodiness, anxiety, speech disorders, isolation, acting out behavior, feeling of inferiority
Adolescence	Ego identity versus role confusion	Ego identity: develops sense of self, personal identity, sexual role identity Role confusion: confusion about sex roles and identity
Early adulthood	Intimacy versus isolation	Intimacy: able to love, commit to another person, create an intimate relationship; economic independence, social independence, moving out, establishing own family Isolation: unable to commit to relationships, lack of intimacy in interpersonal contact, poor impulse control, unable to accept responsibility
Middle age	Generativity versus stagnation	Generativity: productive and creative, cares for others of different ages, concerned with next generation of people Stagnation: self-absorbed, midlife crisis, sense of failure, frustration with aging, sexual inadequacy

POINT TO PONDER

When presented with an age in a question/situation, always think of the person's developmental stage (according to Erikson). This will assist you in identifying the pertinent issues that the nurse should be assessing for at various ages. Look for questions concerning the hospitalized adult or child that point to regression or maladaptation in response to the threat posed by hospitalization.

Erikson's Eight Stages of Psychosocial Development (*continued*)

Age	Developmental Tasks	Exhibited By
Later years	Ego integrity versus despair	Ego integrity: develops new interests, adjusts to decreasing physical abilities, feeling of fulfillment Despair: unable to enjoy future, fears death and illness, lack of satisfaction with life, many regrets

Defense Mechanisms

Mechanism Type	Example	Significance
Compensation	"I'm too busy to get involved in a relationship."	The person is not sure anyone likes her or would like her so she puts her energy into her work.
Conversion reaction	"I can't see, I have gone blind."	The person witnesses a horrible sight or traumatic event and compensates by becoming blind without any physical reason for this blindness.
Denial	"It didn't happen. It is some kind of mistake."	The person is unable to cope with the reality of the situation and believes that some mistake may have been made.
Displacement	"Would you please pick up your room now!" (yelling at child)	The person yelling has been disciplined at work by her boss. She can't yell at the boss, so she waits until she can react (by yelling at someone who is not a threat).
Identification	"Can I have that Madonna shirt, please? Please? Please? Please?"	The person demonstrates an example of hero worship, which is often the reason children try to dress and act like adults and mimic people they like.
Intellectualization	"I need to understand how people develop acute lymphocytic leukemia."	The person may be reacting in response to horrible information such as a diagnosis of a terminal illness.
Projection	"Mommy, you hate me."	The child being punished may say this to her parent. What the child really means is that she (the child) hates her mother, but this is too threatening to say.
Rationalization	"What's the use of studying for the test? The way the teacher asks the questions is not fair."	The person is making an excuse for failing the test for which she didn't bother to study.
Reaction formation	"Is there anything I can do for you? I am available 24 hours a day."	The person wishes to tell the other person how much he dislikes her, but it is much too threatening, so he acts in an overly friendly manner.
Regression	"I wet my bed tonight."	The older sibling reverts to a previous developmental stage in reaction to a stressful situation such as the parents bringing home a new brother or sister.

Defense Mechanisms (*continued*)

Mechanism Type	Example	Significance
Repression	"I don't remember what my attacker looks like, even though I saw him for 10 minutes face-to-face."	The person unconsciously excludes unpleasant memories from her conscious; used in traumatic episodes such as murder, rape, and other violent acts.
Somatization	"I can't take the test today. I am so sick and I have a splitting headache."	This is also known as somatic justification. It is easier to say "I am sick" than it is to say "I am very afraid I'll fail this test."
Sublimation	"I want to be a football player because it is a rough and tumble sport."	The person may have a tendency to violence and physical behavior which is condoned on the football field (and sometimes encouraged).
Suppression	"Don't come home after you take your nursing examination. I am changing the locks on the doors.	"The person who hears this is going to take her licensure examination. In order to take this test and pass it, she goes to the test site and stays focused on the test, while consciously excluding what is happening in her personal life.

Therapeutic Communication Strategies

- A complete understanding of the various therapeutic and nontherapeutic communication techniques is required to better assist you when answering questions. The purpose of communication in nursing care is to establish what the client is saying, understand it, and assist the person to process his or her strengths, areas of growth, and self-concept.

For example: Mr. Jones states, "I am such a failure I can't stand living anymore."

The incorrect responses include telling Mr. Jones that he would be committing a sin, reminding him that those around him would be sad, trivializing his statement by telling him "things will get better," or telling him he shouldn't feel that way. Each of these responses prevents Mr. Jones from responding to the nurse in an open and honest way. This will serve to stop communication between the nurse and Mr. Jones. It implies that his feelings are not of value or of no importance and is considered a communication block. When you select an answer like these, you are offering inappropriate advice and not creating an atmosphere that will allow him to further express his emotions. Avoid any answers that seem even remotely judgmental, and focus on answers that include the communication techniques presented here.

Better (more correct) answers focus on the issue of what makes him feel like a failure, how serious his intentions are (does he have a plan), and how frightening it must be to feel so hopeless and alone.

■ The following are techniques that can be seen in more correct answers than incorrect answers. Using these techniques in any question involving client statements will increase your likelihood of responding correctly. Commit these to memory and look for them in items.

Technique	Response
Silence	The use of silence can be effective because it allows time for reflection and quiet thinking. Nurse: "I know how difficult it is to talk about the accident and how worried you are about your child."
Encouragement	The use of encouragement lets the client know that the nurse wants him to continue with his statements or thoughts. Nurse: "Can you share more information about that?" "Go on." "Please continue with what you were saying."
Acknowledging	This technique gives permission to the client to speak even when it may not be pleasant. Nurse: "You sound angered by your experience." "I can feel your anger." "I notice that you are clenching your fist while speaking about this."
Reflecting	This allows the client to focus on her emotions or response to a situation. Nurse: "How did it make you feel when you were not picked for a team?" "Did you fear you would be left out of the game?"
Restating	The nurse rewords the client's statements to clarify the communication. Nurse: "You sound as though you were frustrated by not being able to get a job after you were fired."
Clarifying	This process attempts to make sure that what the client is communicating is what the nurse is actually hearing. Nurse: "Do I understand that you are angry at everyone in your family except your brother?"
Doubting	This technique can be used in answers to further clarify information that seems unbelievable or impossible. It questions the statement without threatening the client or calling him or her a liar or mistaken. Client: "I spent 100 dollars for my pencil." Nurse: "Isn't that an expensive pencil?"
Observing	In this form of communication, the nurse describes or comments on client/patient behaviors or actions. Nurse: "You have been sitting in the same chair for the last 4 hours staring out the window."
Summarizing	This technique verifies that the nurse is hearing what the client/patient is saying. Nurse: "Do I understand you when you say that you are angry, you mean that you want to kill someone?"

POINT TO PONDER

The use of open-ended questions encourage the client to continue the communication. In the nonemergency situation, it is best to let the client respond to these open-ended questions. Better answers are more likely to be open-ended. The best open-ended questions focus on feelings and reality (look for these).

Nontherapeutic Communication Responses (Blocks to Communication)

Technique	Response
Giving advice	Many responses that offer advice to clients/patients can be considered incorrect. Nurse: "If I were you, I would . . ."
Offering blame	Some responses may attempt to place the blame on something or someone. It is not productive and alienates the person. Nurse "What do you expect if you don't practice safe sex?"
Agreeing with negative attitudes	If a client has committed an act not tolerated by society and expresses remorse or disgust at his actions, do not reinforce his thoughts. Nurse: "Your actions were pretty bad."
Giving false reassurances	This does not help the person feel better or encourage communication. Nurse: "Don't worry about that now; you'll be all right."

Psychosocial/Communication

111

Confidentiality

- Violating client confidentiality is an ethical and legal problem.

- Questions in the NCLEX-PN may describe breaches of client confidentiality in hallways and lunch rooms and on elevators. Every nurse is responsible for protecting a client's right to confidentiality and privacy. Nurses are liable and subject to lawsuits for breach of confidentiality. Defamation of character, libel, slander, and invasion of privacy are all issues related to confidentiality. When presented with these types of situations, always advise the person who is breaching confidentiality to stop at that time, and report the instance to the supervisor.

Managing Anxiety

- Assist the person in identifying the source and cause of the anxiety.

- When talking to the person, comment on behavior such as fist clenching, gritting of teeth, and foot swinging. Validate whether the person is experiencing anxiety and whether they are feeling anxious at that time. Assist clients in identifying and describing what caused the anxiety and how to identify what triggers their emotions. Assure a calm manner during client communications. Organize the environment to decrease activity and stress. Encourage physical activities such as walking, stretching, and swimming. Employ soothing measures such as warm baths, soft music, soft lighting, breathing awareness techniques, and progressive muscle relaxation to assist during episodes of anxiety.

Assessing Appearance and Mood

- Assess facial expression, gait, movement, dress, orientation, speech, attitude, client statements as to feelings, the nurse–client interaction, the appropriateness of affect, thought processes, thought content, feelings of worthlessness, perceptions, intellectual functioning, memory, insight, judgment, and danger to self or to others.

Distinguishing Between Delusions, Illusions, and Hallucinations

- *Delusions* are false, fixed beliefs that cannot be changed with reasoning: delusions of grandeur "I am God"; delusions of persecution ("Everybody is trying to hurt me.") *Hallucinations* are imaginary sense experiences which are not shared by anyone else (seeing things that are not there, hearing voices, smelling something not present). *Illusions* are misinterpretations of what is being seen (eg, water on the highway on a hot, sunny day).

Crisis Intervention

MANAGEMENT FOR THE HALLUCINATING CLIENT

- Look for answers that:
  State the facts if a situation presents with the client appearing confused or frightened.
  > Nurse: "You look frightened."
  > Nurse: "I heard you talking to someone."
  Discredit the hallucination without discrediting the person.
  > Nurse: "What do the voices *that you hear* say to you?"
  > Nurse: "*Do you see* the person as we are talking?"

Depression and Suicide

- Depressed clients are most suicidal when they begin to feel better and are able to gather up strength to commit the act.

Suicide Precautions

- Inform clients that they are on suicide precautions.
- Clients must always be in the view of staff.
- Clients may or may not be able to use the bathroom alone.
- Make sure clients swallow all medications.
- Keep all potentially dangerous personal possessions locked up.
- When serving meals and snacks, don't allow sharp utensils to be used.
- When assessing crisis situations and suicidal periods, look for direct responses such as:
  "Do you feel like hurting yourself now?"
  "Have you thought about taking your own life?"
  "Do you have a plan on how you will kill yourself?"

Managing Violent Behavior

- When violence occurs, the response must be immediate, and the client must be informed that violence is not an acceptable course of action.
- Remove all persons at risk for injury.
- Notify security personnel and other units.
- Talk to the client quietly and firmly.
- Lead the client away from the cause of agitation.
- Encourage the client to calm down.
- If the client poses a threat to self or others, use physical restraint with order.
- Documentation must include information about why the form of restraint was necessary, and that the ADLs were met throughout the time of restraint.

Abuse of Children and Adults

- Assess for physical evidence of abuse (look for patterns of bruises/injuries).
- Be alert to conflicting stories about the injury (look for blaming the injury on the person injured).
- Parents may attempt to get their child discharged when confronted with suspected abuse.
- Abuse must be reported if the client is a child, an elder, or mentally incapacitated.
- If the adult client insists on returning to the home, help to develop an escape plan and a place to go.

Initial Management for Rape Trauma Syndrome

- Ensure the client's privacy during the interview.
- Remain with the client.
- Help the client retell the event in her own words.
- Gather data and evidence.
- Assist with the physical examination as indicated.

Psychosocial/Communication

- Reassure victims that they are not to blame.
- Help the client notify family/significant other.
- After physical examination, help the client to bathe and change clothes, and have someone bring in fresh clothes.

Posttraumatic Stress Disorder (PTSD)

- PTSD can follow wars, natural catastrophes, attacks, rape, muggings, or incest.
- Signs and symptoms include flashbacks, poor interpersonal relationships, inability to function at home or work, and severe anxiety.
- Use a nonjudgmental approach while encouraging the client to express feelings during periods of stress.

Management of Sexually Provocative Behavior

- Limit sexual activity at all times and be direct.
  Nurse: "Mr. Flynn, that type of behavior is inappropriate here."
  Nurse: "Mr. Flynn, please stop exposing your genitals in the hallway."
  Nurse: "Mr. Flynn, please take your hand off of me immediately."

ELDER CARE ISSUES AND MANAGEMENT CONSIDERATIONS

Integumentary System

- Decreased sweat/sebaceous gland function, resulting in dry skin.
  Less frequent bathing required; avoid drying soaps.
  Use moisturizers.
- Decreased thickness of skin/subcutaneous layer.
  More prone to injury, pressure sores, skin infections, skin tears, and heat loss/hypothermia.
  Avoid overuse of tape for dressings; consider using Montgomery straps.
  Keep environment warm.
  Avoid drafts and keep appropriately covered.
- Increased fragility of blood vessels.
  More prone to bruising

Exposure to Sunlight

- More prone to skin cancers.
  Assess areas exposed to sun.
  Note areas of skin with senile keratosis (raised brown patches).
  Assess for lesions that could be basal or squamous cell carcinomas.

Management Considerations

- Assess skin for evidence of redness, breakdowns, and infections.
- Reduce bathing to once or twice per week unless otherwise needed.
- Treat wounds as ordered; note and record changes daily.
- Provide appropriate foot care and skin care of lower extremities to prevent breakdown and infections.
- Keep environment warm.
- Provide adequate clothing for the environment.
- Keep out of drafty areas and monitor closely when outside.

Respiratory System

- Increased rigidity of alveoli.

  Changes in lung function may include chronic lung disease (emphysema and bronchitis).

- Decreased number and effectiveness of cilia.

  More likely to react to dust, pollens, and powder.

  Avoid exposure to environmental irritants in older adults.

  Avoid crowds to prevent or decrease incidence of pneumonia and influenza (flu).

  Reactivation of old tuberculosis.

  Note complaints of sputum production, lethargy, weight loss, and fatigue.

Management Considerations

- Assess baseline respiratory patterns.

- Teach client how to improve breathing ability by using the abdominal muscles and intercostals, and splinting when appropriate.

- Space activities to avoid overtiring clients.

- Assist in clearing secretions by teaching and encouraging coughing, deep breathing exercises, postural drainage, and use of incentive spirometry as ordered.

- Assess for episodes of shortness of breath, use of secondary accessory muscles, and increased respiratory rate during activity.

- Teach client to report all respiratory problems when they develop.

Musculoskeletal System

- Decreased amount of calcium in bones.

  Prone to develop osteoporosis, decreased height, vertebral collapse, and fractures.

  More likely to develop degenerative arthritis, rheumatoid arthritis, and bursitis.

Management Considerations

- Assess current and past activity levels.

- Develop a regular exercise routine for clients.

- Promote active and passive range of motion excercises for clients on bedrest or otherwise restricted.

- Position client in good alignment in bed to prevent development of contractures and muscle atrophy.

- Provide assistance during ambulation as necessary. Use appropriate adaptive devices, such as gait belts, to assist with ambulation.

- Teach client how to use canes, walkers, and other assistive devices.

- Use the least amount of restraint ordered for the client to minimize restrictions in activity.

Cardiovascular System

- Changes in the heart muscle, leading to decreased cardiac output.

  Prone to coronary artery disease such as angina, valve disease, congestive heart failure, and dysrhythmias.

  Cardiomegaly (enlarged heart) occurs to compensate for decreasing effectiveness of the heart muscle.

- Thickening of blood vessels leading to atherosclerosis.
  Prone to hypertension and changes associated with increased blood pressure.
  Prone to varicose veins and thrombophlebitis.
  Peripheral edema.

Management Considerations

- Monitor client's baseline vital signs for activities and teach when to discontinue if problems arise.
- Instruct client to report episodes of lightheadedness, dizziness, chest pain, palpations, or shortness of breath during activities.
- Monitor vital signs and peripheral pulses during activity periods and cease activity if client offers any of the above complaints.
- Report complaints of lightheadedness, dizziness, chest pain, palpations, or shortness of breath during activities or at rest immediately.

Hematologic System

- Decreased blood cell production.
  Prone to anemias and leukemias.
- Decreased production of lymphocytes.
  Increased likelihood of infections.

Management Considerations

- Assess baseline vital signs.
- Encourage avoiding exposure to large crowds and environmental extremes.
- Monitor client during transfusions and report any untoward events or reactions.
- Avoid activities that can promote infections.
- Employ neutropenic precautions as ordered.

Gastrointestinal System

- Decreased effectiveness of tastebuds and olfactory nerve (smell).
- Diminished gag reflex.
  More likely to develop aspiration pneumonia and obstruction (choking) on food.
- Decreased peristalsis.
  Prone to constipation, bowel pattern changes, and fecal impactions.
  May develop hemorrhoids with straining to stool/defecate.

Management Considerations

- Nutritional management:
  Encourage proper nutrition, including well-balanced diet with vitamin supplements of A, C, D, E, K, and B complex.
  Weigh regularly, noting changes (at least weekly).
  Prepare meals in appealing ways.
  Offer meals in groups to provide for socialization during mealtime.
  Assess for food preferences.
  Assess skin, hair, nails, and laboratory values (albumin and protein) to monitor effectiveness of nutritional intake.

Record amount of intake and food types.

Prepare a meal plan for home care clients (consult with dietitian).

Monitor intake and output for fluid intake.

Keep fluids at bedside and near client at all times; note fluid preferences.

Note swallowing difficulty, and report.

Keep dentures easily accessible for use during the day; clean dentures daily.

Assist clients with swallowing difficulty to keep head upright and neck slightly flexed to enhance swallowing.

Provide verbal cuing of clients during mealtimes.

Provide food supplements as ordered.

Monitor for aspiration and episodes of choking; report to physician.

Administer tube feedings as ordered.

Note problems with teeth and mucous membranes, and report.

Provide proper oral hygiene before and after meals.

- Bowel management:

  Determine current and past bowel patterns.

  Encourage increasing physical acitivity.

  Encourage increasing fluid intake to 2000 to 3000 mL per day (unless contraindicated).

  Encourage high-fiber diet with high roughage.

  Administer stool softeners and laxatives per order, and maintain schedule.

  Develop regular toileting schedule, and promote privacy.

  Proper skin care during episodes of loose stools.

Genitourinary System

- Decreased muscle tone of bladder and pelvic organs/muscles.

  Prone to incontinence.

  Prone to urinary tract infections.

- Increased prostate size.

  Prone to urinary retention and bladder distention.

  Prone to incontinence.

- Decreased number of nephrons.

  Less reserve capacity, resulting in possibility of developing renal failure and chronic renal insufficiency.

Management Considerations

- Assess current and past urinary elimination patterns.

- Note, record, and report episodes of urinary incontinence to establish patterns and frequency.

- Provide for regular toileting schedule and opportunities to use commodes and urinals to decrease episodes of incontinence.

- Teach Kegel exercises (pelvic muscle floor strengthening exercises) to promote decreased stress incontinence in women, and post-prostatectomy in men.

- Provide appropriate skin care for incontinent clients and apply incontinent pads as directed.

- Provide proper catheter care as ordered for clients with indwelling catheters.

- Provide emotional support to client and family/significant others of clients experiencing episodes of urinary incontinence.
- Increase physical activity.

Neurologic System

- Decreased number of brain cells.
  Prone to dementing processes including Alzheimer's disease.
  Decreasing reflexes and motor responses, resulting in diseases such as Parkinson's disease, senile ataxia (more difficulty walking), slower responses and reaction time to potential problems, and falls.
- Changes in blood vessels in the brain and circulation to the brain.
  Increased incidence of transient ischemic attacks and cerebrovascular accidents.

Management Considerations

- Prevent falls: assess for potential; reduce environmental risks such as maintaining well-lit hallways and bathroom areas (especially at night).
- Maintain bed in lowest position.
- Move at a comfortable pace; do not rush.
- Encourage proper footwear with nonskid soles, no throw rugs in house; keep low objects away from walking areas.
- In Alzheimer's disease, clients may not know who they are, where they are, or the time/date.

Therapeutic Management of Alzheimer's

- For wandering behavior, the client must be kept in a safe, supervised environment.
- Decrease access to dangerous areas, lock exits, and remember that wandering is a stress reliever for some clients.
- Encourage group activities in place of wandering activities.
- Have finger foods available for wanderers who are unable to sit long enough for meals.
- People with organic impairments will have short-term memory lapses and difficulty recalling a story. They may confabulate (make up) a story.
- People in delirium states will also have short-term memory problems. High levels of anxiety will negatively affect this type of assessment.
- Provide activities to stimulate the client and decrease the possibility of sensory deprivation.
- Note, record, and report episodes of confusion and disorientation.
- Encourage group activities such as reminiscence therapy, reality orientation groups, and socialization.
- Provide a safe environment for wandering clients by keeping doors closed and locked as necessary, and keeping all medications, cleansers, and dangerous items locked away.
- Keep small, loose items to a minimum in the environment.

Integumentary System

Sunburn

- Use PABA-free sunscreen for infants and children.
- Cover infants with hats and long-sleeved garments.

Respiratory System

Breathing Patterns

- Newborn breathing rate is approximately 40 breaths per minute.
- Wheezes: high-pitched, musical sounds heard in large airway narrowing such as asthma, bronchitis, and chronic lung disease. Sudden cessation of wheezes may indicate airway closure and is a medical emergency.
- Stridor: crowing sound indicative of acute airway narrowing.

Epiglottitis

- Symptoms develop suddenly.
- Child presents with drooling, inability to swallow, croaking sound with breathing. Child sits forward with mouth open and "looks sick."

SAFETY TIP

Emergency equipment at bedside should include an intubation kit.

Keep fingers and items out of mouth.

Bronchiolitis

- Frequently occurs soon after an upper respiratory infection or after exposure to respiratory syncytial virus (RSV).
- Symptoms include nasal discharges and congestion, wheezing, and increased respiratory rate.

MANAGEMENT

- Maintain high humidity and keep the client hydrated (make sure he or she can drink if fluids are administered by mouth).
- Client will be put on respiratory precautions.

Tonsillectomy

- Tonsils are removed if there is a history of recurrent or chronic infections.
- The client will have difficulty swallowing postoperatively.

Croup

- Likely complaints and findings include a barking cough, rib retractions, stridor, an increased breathing rate, and fever (102°F or above).

MANAGEMENT

- Croup tent (cool mist).
- Humidified oxygen per order.
- IV fluids may be ordered for dehydration and improvement of circulation.

SAFETY TIP

Assess for progressive shortness of breath.

Cystic Fibrosis

- This genetic disorder occurs in newborns and affects the lungs, liver, and pancreas.
- Foul-smelling stools may be noted.
- Infant may be diagnosed with failure to thrive.
- Diet: high-protein, high-carbohydrate, low-fat, *increased salt* in summer.
- Respiratory infections are common.

Sudden Infant Death Syndrome (SIDS)

- This condition results in the sudden death of an infant under one year of age.
- The infant may be placed on an apnea monitor at home.

SAFETY TIP

Infants and children should be put to sleep on their back or either side, but not prone. Sleeping on the back has reduced deaths by more than 30%.

Cardiovascular System

Congenital Heart Disorders in Children

- Infants may present with failure to thrive (FTT), have difficulty feeding, and can become cyanotic when crying.

- Older children are very small for age and may feel better in the squat position.
- Monitor for development of congestive heart failure (CHF).

TETRALOGY OF FALLOT (SEVERE DEFECT)

- Child will squat to obtain relief from cyanotic spells; usually has cyanosis and fatigue.
- Managed through surgical correction of defect.

PATENT DUCTUS ARTERIOSUS

- Occurs in premature infants; detected by poor feeding patterns and recurrent respiratory infections.

ATRIAL SEPTAL DEFECT

- Enlarged heart and a heart murmur frequently detected.

VENTRICULOSEPTAL DEFECT

- Shortness of breath, increased weight (much more than expected), and signs and symptoms of CHF in severe cases.

PULMONARY STENOSIS

- CHF in advanced stage.

AORTIC STENOSIS

- Chest pain may occur with exercise.

COARCTATION OF AORTA

- Blood pressure differences found in upper and lower extremities; may have headache or lightheadedness.

RHEUMATIC FEVER

- Occurs after strep infection (group A beta hemolytic strep).
- Make sure clients comply with the antibiotic regimen for 10 days to eliminate strep infection.
- Heart valve damage can occur when infection is not treated promptly.

Hematologic System

Hemophilia

- Children treated for hemophilia in the early 1980s exposed to HIV may contract AIDS.
- Teach parents to provide care after any injury and to assess carefully for hematomas.

Lead Poisoning

- A toxic reaction is caused by eating lead paint or being exposed to high levels of environmental lead.
- Levels may be lowered by injection of chelating agents.

POINT TO PONDER

Allow children to express anger over injections (eg, have them pound clay). Make sure that no procedures occur in their bedroom, which must be considered the "safe room."

POINT TO PONDER

Sickle cell anemia may cause cerebrovascular accidents (strokes) even in young children.

Sickle Cell Anemia

- An inherited genetic disorder (with the highest incidence in black populations) that causes blood cells to become more rigid and thick, which blocks circulation in the capillaries.
- Parents should be taught to report even minor infections and to keep the child well hydrated.
- During crisis periods, hydration, analgesics, bedrest, and heat applications to the areas affected will provide relief.
- Look for complaints of pain or throbbing in affected areas.

Thalassemias

- Genetic disorder seen in children and adults of Mediterranean and African-American heritage.
- May require blood transfusions or splenectomy.
- Thalassemia major (Cooley's anemia) clients usually die in the 16-to-24 age group due to iron overload.

Leukemia

- The most frequently occurring leukemia in children is known as acute lymphocytic leukemia.
- All leukemias can lead to complaints of fatigue, frequent infections, bruising, bleeding, and bone pain.
- Managed with chemotherapy and bone marrow transplants. Assess for usual side effects such as nausea and vomiting, loss of hair (alopecia), and fungal infections in mouth and throat (thrush).
- Assist client and parents in coping with the complicated nature of the disease and treatments.

Gastrointestinal System

Failure to Thrive (FTT) (Nonorganic)

- Can occur from infancy to teen years; presents with malnourished state, poor growth patterns, and eating disorders.
- Child may appear withdrawn and apathetic toward new situations and strange people.
- Assist children in developing appropriate eating habits; help parents to encourage interactions with child.

POINT TO PONDER

Remember the Cs of eating: Coughing, Choking, Cyanosis.

Pyloric Stenosis

- This condition may have a family history; affects newborns, males, and first child.
- Symptoms include projectile vomiting and FTT.
- Management includes surgical intervention and providing the infant with a thickened formula for better digestion.

Cellophane Tape Test

- Cellophane tape is placed on anal opening to detect pinworms.
- Common in children and usually performed in the early morning.

Genitourinary System

Acute Glomerulonephritis/Nephrotic Syndrome

- In AGN children have oliguria (scant urine production), edema, and hypertension.
- Nephrotic syndrome presents with edema throughout the body (especially in the eye area), increased blood pressure, and protein in the urine.
- AGN management includes antibiotics, lowering serum potassium, and dialysis.

Musculoskeletal System

Congenital Hip Dysplasia

- The gluteal folds will appear unequal in infants.
- When the hips are moved, a clicking sound is heard (Ortolani's click).
- Managed by placing the child in a spica cast or, in mild forms, by double diapering the infant.

Scoliosis

- Brace surgery may be required.
- Harrison rods may be used to surgically correct the condition.
- If placed in a Milwaukee brace, the child will be in it 23 hours per day.
- Child has to cope with significant alteration in body image.

Neurologic System

Seizure Disorders

- Atonic (drop attacks in infants and children) and myoclonic seizures:
  Signs and symptoms of these can include sudden loss of consciousness for a short time or sudden muscle jerking.
  Consult physician for follow-up (potential brain damage).
- Absence (petit mal):
  Frequently begin around age 4 to puberty and may appear as "daydreaming."
  Advise parents to follow up if children have episodes of memory loss lasting for several seconds to several minutes.

Hydrocephalus in Infants

- Occurs when there is a decrease in the outflow of cerebrospinal fluid (CSF) from the brain, which increases pressure within the brain and leads to an enlarged head, increased circumference, bulging fontnels in infants, and headaches.
- Keep the infant's head supported at all times.

POINT TO PONDER

In children especially, look for AGN preceded by strep throat or bacterial infection.

POINT TO PONDER

Never force the mouth open, attempt to restrain the tongue, or give anything by mouth during a seizure.

Down Syndrome and Trisomy

■ These are genetic disorders that create an extra chromosome.

Spina Bifida and Meningocele

■ Conditions in which the cord, meninges, spinal fluid, and nerves (or just the cord and meninges) are found outside the spinal column, which can cause paraplegia and poor bladder or bowel control.

■ Hold infant in sitting position when feeding.

■ When lying, keep infant on side (supported) or on abdomen.

■ Requires surgical correction.

Special Senses

Cleft Lip and Cleft Palate

■ Repaired surgically several weeks after birth.

■ A soft nipple is recommended for feeding infants.

■ Child may be placed in elbow restraints to prevent damage to sutures.

Strabismus

■ Known as "lazy eye"; occurs as a result of eye muscle weakness.

Otitis Media

■ Occurs most frequently in children under the age of 3.

■ Child may have a shortened eustachian tube that is angled at a more horizontal level.

Developmental Milestones ▶

■ Expect the following to be important milestone in each age group.

■ 1 month:
  Reflexes present (Moro, suck, tonic neck)
  Holds head up briefly
  Needs support for head when held

■ 2 months:
  Reflexes still present
  Lifts head when on stomach
  Can support head when being held briefly

■ 3 months:
  Reflexes begin to fade
  Holds head up when being held
  Holds head up when on stomach
  Can sit briefly with supports
  Responds to mother's voice with cooing

- 4 months:
  Can move head in all directions when being held
  Kicks; moves arms and legs with purpose
  May roll from stomach to back
  Sits briefly without support

- 5 months:
  Can sit with little support
  Rolls from stomach to back
  Can support self when held in standing position
  Babbles

- 6 months:
  Pulls self to sitting position
  Can sit in an infant chair with little support
  Crawls

- 7 months:
  Pulls self to sitting position
  Stands and supports weight when held
  Crawls without difficulty

- 8 months:
  Supports self alone briefly
  Sits alone and moves to creeping position

- 9 months:
  Stands alone briefly
  Cruises from one piece of furniture to another
  Pulls self to standing position

- 10 months:
  Walks briefly while holding onto something
  Creeps rapidly
  Understands spoken language

- 11 to 12 months:
  Walks alone
  Goes from standing to sitting

- 12 to 15 months:
  Walks alone for great distances
  Begins to jump
  Crawls up stairs
  Begins to speak

- 15 to 18 months:
  Can walk pulling objects
  Creeps down stairs
  Pushes large objects around

- 18 to 24 months:
  Runs well
  Jumps
  Walks up and down stairs
  Speaks in short sentences

- 2 to 3 years:
  Throws ball
  Stands on tiptoes
  Steady on feet

- 3 to 5 years:
    Walks backward
    Walks up and down stairs alternating feet
    Pedals tricycle
    Begins to skip
    Can play games that require skill in running
- 5 to 10 years:
    Can skate or run with skill
    Ties shoe laces
    Dresses self
    Bathes self
    Swims
    Jumps rope
    Develops skills with basketball, football, baseball
- 10 to 12 years:
    Early puberty begins
- Adolescents:
    Puberty begins for girls from age 11 to 13 years
    Puberty begins for boys from age 13 to 15 years

Appropriate Toy Selections for Infants ▶ and Children

- 1 to 3 months:
    Mobile above crib
    Music
    Large, bright objects
    Soft stuffed animals
- 3 to 6 months:
    Rattle
    Music
    Crib gym
    Toys that make noise when moved
- 6 to 9 months:
    Household objects that make noise and can be dropped
    Pots and pans
    Teething rings
    Bath toys
    Mirror
    Ball (soft and noisy)
- 9 to 12 months:
    More pots and pans
    Mirror (nonbreakable)
    Books (cloth or paper)
    Jack-in-the-box
    Musical toys
- 12 to 15 months:
    Large plastic toys
    Blocks
    Stacking items
    Own spoon and cup
    Toys to push and pull

- 15 to 18 months:
    Large riding toys
    Shopping cart
    Play lawn mower
    Push–pull toys
    Plastic slide
    Large cardboard boxes
- 18 months to 2 years:
    Toys with different shapes to fit together
    Wooden train
    Large cars and trucks
    Finger paint
    Water toys
- 2 year to 3 years:
    Wagon
    Tricycle
    Clay
    Crayons and paper
    Toy telephone
    Household toys (broom, vacuum cleaner, mop)
    Puzzles
- 3 to 5 years:
    Records and tapes
    Books
    Playground toys
    Sandbox
    Modeling clay
    Simple games
    Dolls, doll houses, stuffed animals
    Dress up clothes and shoes
    Simple card games
    Bicycle
    Scissors and paper
    Puzzles
    Ball games and group play
- 5 to 12 years:
    Skates (ice and roller)
    Games (tag, baseball, soccer)
    Simple carpentry tools
    Coloring books, crayons, markers
    Balls
    Games (checkers, dominoes, basketball, and football)
    Swimming
    Crafts
    Musical instruments
    Models

Reproductive Disorders in Females ▶

Anatomy	Problems
Vulva	Lesions (such as herpes lesions/vesicles and cysts), warts
Urethra	Urethritis (gonococcal and nongonococcal)
Vagina	Various types of infections
Cervix	Inflammation, dysplasia, and carcinoma
Uterus	Fibroids and carcinoma

Hysterectomy

- Surgical removal of the uterus, ovaries, tubes, and lymph node dissection as part of treatment of carcinoma.
- Data collection of cervical carcinoma include abnormal vaginal bleeding, abdominal distention, back pain, vaginal discharge, or a feeling of pressure.
- Postoperative:
    Counsel on alteration in body image and the grief response; encourage attendance at support groups.
    Limit activities such as sexual intercourse, riding horses, skiing, or heavy lifting for 6 weeks.
    Teach about signs and symptoms of surgical menopause such as hot flashes, insomnia, depression, irritability, and increased perspiration.

Premenstrual Syndrome

- Lower salt, sugar, caffeine, chocolate, alcohol, and red meat intake.

Syphilis (Treponema pallidum)

- Serologic tests (VDRL, FTA-ABS IgM).
- Early stage: chancre (painless) and general malaise for 6 weeks.
- Secondary stage: development of fine rash on palms and soles, venereal warts, weight loss, conjunctivitis, alopecia.
- Tertiary stage: cardiovascular, dementia, and ataxia.
- Syphilis during pregnancy may cause spontaneous abortion or birth of a baby that is small for gestational age.

Neisseria gonorrhoeae

- Female: early symptoms range from none to mild discharge which may result in pelvic inflammatory disease (PID).
- Male: pain with heavy greenish-yellow discharge/urethritis.

Chlamydia trachomatis

- Signs and symptoms include a thin mucopurulent discharge, which may present complications to the neonate such as stillbirth, conjunctivitis, and pneumonia.
- Managed using erythromycin ointment.

Genital Herpes (HSV II)

- Data collection: assess for painful blisters that rupture and form crusts.

- Active lesions prior to delivery indicate the need for cesarean section.
- Medication used for treatment is acyclovir.

Trichomonas vaginalis

- Data collection focuses on production of a profuse, yellow-green, frothy, odorous discharge.
- Management: all oral medications are contraindicated in the first trimester of pregnancy.
- Nonpregnant clients are treated with metronidazole (Flagyl).

Breast Cancer

- Increased incidence in postmenopausal women.
- Data collection includes assessing for painless lump(s) (hard and immovable); nipple inversion/discharge; breast tenderness; and dimpling, puckering, or retraction of breast.
- Postoperative management: relieve anxiety; assist in adapting to body image changes and sexuality.
- Recommend support groups (eg, Reach to Recovery).
- Restore ROM to arm.
- No restrictive garments, blood pressure measurement, or IVs on affected side. Teach signs and symptoms of infection.

Reproductive Disorders in Males

Anatomy	Problems
Penis	Hypospadias (urethral opening on the ventral side of penis), epispadias (urethral opening on dorsal side of the penis)
Scrotum	Hydrocele, hematocele, cryptorchidism (undescended testicle)
Urethra	Urethritis (gonococcal and nongonococcal)
Prostate	Inflammation, benign prostatic hypertrophy, and cancer

Prostatic Hypertrophy

- Usually males over age 50 develop benign prostatic hypertrophy or prostate cancer.
- Lab test: prostate-specific antigen (PSA) positive for cancer.
- Later signs include intermittent stream, painful urination, dribbling, overflow or paradoxical incontinence, and nocturia.
- Surgical interventions: transurethral resection of prostate (TURP); most common procedure with removal of the prostate via cystoscope.
- Postoperative care:
  Catheter care: three-way Foley catheter, 30-cc balloon. Keep catheter patent by irrigating for clots.
  Expect that urine will be bright red immediately postoperatively, then will turn pink to straw-colored in 24 hours.
- Client education:
  No heavy lifting or driving for 6 weeks.
  Intake of 8 to 10 glasses of water per day.

POINT TO PONDER

Perform self breast exam 1 week after menstrual period. After menopause, same day each month. Screening mammogram baseline: 35 to 50 years old, every 1 to 2 years; over 50 years old, every year.

POINT TO PONDER

Earliest warning sign is a decrease in the urinary stream and hesitancy in beginning urination.

Teach client that urine may contain small amounts of blood at times, and may be pink.

Teach pelvic floor muscle training to decrease incontinence.

No rectal temps for 4 to 6 weeks.

Avoid constipation and straining at the stool; encourage use of stool softeners and high-fiber diet.

No sex for 6 weeks.

Birth Control Methods and Types ▶

Methods	Examples
Natural family planning	Billing's method (cervical mucus monitoring)
Hormonal	Oral contraceptives, Norplant, Depo-Provera
Barrier methods	Diaphragm and spermicide, cervical cap, vaginal sponge, condoms
Other methods	IUD, tubal ligation, vasectomy

Pregnancy

Data Collection

- Estimated date of confinement (EDC)
- Estimated date of delivery (EDD)
- Naegele's rule: add 7 days to the first day of the last menstrual period and subtract 3 months.

Signs of Pregnancy

- Presumptive: amenorrhea, nausea and vomiting, urinary frequency, fatigue, breast changes.
- Probable: Goodell's sign (softening of the cervix), Chadwick's sign (bluing of the vaginal mucosa), ballottement (palpation of uterine contents), positive pregnancy test, quickening (maternal perception of fetal movement).
- Positive (diagnostic): fetal heart rate by Doppler (10 to 12 weeks), fetoscope (fetal heart rate heard by 16 to 20 weeks), fetal movement felt by examiner, ultrasonography to detect the presence of a fetus, fetal electrocardiography.

Diagnostic Tests

Ultrasound

- Performed to determine gestational age, fetal growth, fetal size, multiple pregnancy, fetal position, and diagnosis of congenital anomalies and bleeding disorders.

Electronic Fetal Heart Rate Monitoring (EFM)

- Helps to determine fetal well-being or high risk.

Amniocentesis

- Assesses for genetic defects (Down syndrome, Tay–Sachs, sickle cell, thalassemia, and neural tube defect).
- Performed at 15 to 18 weeks.

Prenatal Data Collection

- Family history for diabetes, heart disease, hypertension, and cancer.
- Past gynecologic disorders and diseases (eg, PID).
- Previous pregnancies and deliveries.
- Partner.

Common Problems in Pregnancy

Respiratory

- Nasal stuffiness, dyspnea (shortness of breath), increased rate of breathing (to compensate for decreased ability to breathe deeply).
- Recommendations: saline drops for nose, add pillows when in bed, and continue to exercise moderately.

Cardiovascular

- Increased fluid retention (ankle edema), anemia, supine hypotension, varicose veins.
- Recommendations: elevate feet, lie in left lateral position, and moderate exercise.

Gastrointestinal

- Nausea/vomiting (morning sickness) reflux, heartburn, constipation, pica.
- Recommendations: frequent (small) meals, crackers, increase fluids and fiber, antacids.

Genitourinary

- Risk for UTI, frequency.
- Recommendations: increase fluid intake, Kegel exercises, know UTI signs and symptoms.

Endocrine

- Weight gain (2–4 lb first trimester and 1 lb per week for other 28 weeks), Braxton–Hicks sign.
- Recommendations: maintain proper posture and body mechanics, pelvic tilt/rock exercises.

Musculoskeletal

- Waddling gait, lower back pain, muscle spasms, diastasis recti.
- Recommendations: encourage calcium intake (dairy products), flat (nonskid surface) shoes, leg exercises, pelvic floor/muscle exercises.

Integumentary

- Striae gravidarum (stretch marks); chloasma ("mask of pregnancy"— erythema around the nose and cheeks).
- Breasts develop appearance of Montgomery tubercles (sebaceous glands on areola); darkening of areola.
- Recommendations: reinforce that pigmentation will fade.

Specific Disorders in Pregnancy

Gestational/Juvenile Diabetes (Disorder During Pregnancy)

- Baby weighs over 4000 grams (macrosomia).
- Difficult labor.
- Hydramnios and pregnancy-induced hypertension (PIH).
- Premature labor and delivery.
- Baby does best when delivered before 36 weeks.
- Infant shows signs of weight loss, glycosuria, and elevated blood sugar.

Pregnancy-induced Hypertension (PIH) (Preeclampsia and Eclampsia)

- Appears after the 20th week and up to 48 hours after delivery.
- Mild: 140/90 mm Hg; protein found in urine and weight gain.
- Severe: 160/110 mm Hg (on two readings within 6 hours); above symptoms and signs plus puffiness of hands and face and significant weight gain.
- Danger signals: hypertension, severe edema, proteinuria, visual disturbances, intractable headaches, and convulsions.

MANAGEMENT

- Mild:
    Bedrest at home; teach warning signs and symptoms.
- Severe:
    Requires hospitalization.
    Monitor blood pressure evaluation QID.
    Intake and output (check for protein in urine).
    Daily weight.
    Monitor for signs and symptoms of labor or seizures.
    Nutrition: high-protein, normal-salt diet.
    Medications: magnesium sulfate ($MgSO_4$) if ordered.
    Antidote: have calcium gluconate at bedside.
- Decrease environmental stimuli.
- For fetus: nonstress test (NST) to assess well being.
- Betamethasone is given to mature a baby's lungs in case of premature delivery.

Supine Hypotension Syndrome in Pregnancy

- The weight of large uterus puts pressure on vena cava.
- Suggest that the client lie on her left side to take pressure off vena cava. Instruct the client to never lie flat on her back.

First-trimester Bleeding

- Abortions: spontaneous; client complains of pain and cramping.
- Management: bedrest, evaluate for shock, prepare for vacuum and curettage.

POINT TO PONDER

Triad of symptoms: hypertension, edema, proteinuria (sign of most advanced stage).

POINT TO PONDER

Gain of 3 to 4 or more pounds per week in last trimester is abnormal and can indicate severe problems.

POINT TO PONDER

Monitor for HELLP syndrome: Hematologic studies, Elevated hemolysis, Liver enzymes, Low Platelets.

Monitor bleeding, clots, and tissue passage; save and count pads, note type of bleeding (bright red, brown, clots). Report and record findings.

- Emotional response: look for grief/anxiety.
- If blood type is Rh negative, RhoGAM is ordered.

Third-trimester Bleeding

- Placenta previa:
    Note uterine bleeding: painless; bright red; monitor for shock and hypovolemia.
    Prepare for cesarean section.
- Abruptio placentae:
    The uterus becomes "boardlike" (hypertonic); client experiences mild to severe pain and uterine bleeding.
    Report immediately, estimate blood loss, and monitor for fetal heart rate and shock.
    Prepare for cesarean section.
    Complication: hemorrhage (bleeding greater than 500 mL in 24 hours).

Hemolytic Disease in Pregnancy

- Rh negative and ABO incompatibility (if mother is Rh negative, father is Rh positive, and baby is Rh positive, mother must get RhoGAM within 72 hours after delivery).
- Assess infant for jaundice within first 24 hours after delivery.
- Phototherapy:
    Protect eyes (black mask).
    No Vaseline (prevent burns).
    Check for signs and symptoms of dehydration.

Labor and Delivery

Signs and Symptoms of Impending Labor

- Lightening: dropping of presenting part into pelvis 2 to 3 weeks prior to delivery.
- Braxton–Hicks: false labor contractions.
- Weight loss: usually 1 to 3 pounds.
- Energy level: increases.
- Cervix: softening/effacement.
- Spontaneous rupture of membranes (SROM): may occur 12 to 24 hours prior to labor.

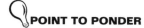

POINT TO PONDER

Do pad count and estimate size and amount of clots.

Signs and Symptoms of True Labor

- Contractions occur with regularity.
- Contractions increase in intensity and duration.
- Contractions start at the back and radiate to the front.
- Contractions intensify while walking.
- Discharge of mucus plug and bloody show.
- Effacement and dilatation of cervix.

Stages/Phases of Labor and Delivery

Stage 1

LATENT PHASE

- Dilatation and effacement: 0 to 3 cm.
- Frequency: contractions start every 20 to 25 minutes, increase to 5 minutes apart, last 30 to 45 seconds, and are of mild intensity.

ACTIVE PHASE

- Dilatation: 3 to 7 cm.
- Frequency: contractions start every 3 to 5 minutes, last 30 to 45 seconds, and are of moderate intensity.

ACTIVE PHASE/TRANSITION

- Dilatation: 8 to 10 cm.
- Frequency: contractions start every 2 minutes; last 60 to 90 seconds, and are of strong intensity.

Stage 2

EXPULSION

- Dilatation: fully dilated.
- Frequency: contractions start every 2 to 3 minutes, 60 seconds' duration, and of strong intensity.
- Pushing: three to four per contraction.

INFANT STATUS

- Normal fetal heart rate (FHR) is 120 to 160 beats per minute.
- Late decelerations: fetal hypoxia–bradycardia (defined as FHR less than 100 beats per minute or a 20-beat-per-minute drop), decrease in beat-to-beat variability, tachycardia (defined as FHR greater than 160 beats per minute).

Stage 3

PLACENTAL (FROM DELIVERY OF THE BABY TO DELIVERY OF THE PLACENTA)

- Data collection focus is on fundus, lochia production, and vital signs.

Stage 4

RECOVERY

- Monitor lochia: color, amount, character, and odor.
  Types: rubra (bright red) from days 1 to 3; serosa (brown) from days 4 to 10; alba (white) from days 11 to 21.

■ Perineal care: check episiotomy for edema/hematomas/stitches. Use of ice, if ordered, can be followed by sitz baths and topical medications for pain. Check for hemorrhoids.

Mother due to void within 8 hours after delivery.

Newborn/Infant Assessment and Management

■ Normal respiratory rate is 30 to 60 breaths per minute.

■ Blood pressure at birth is 80 to 90 systole, 40 to 45 diastole (mm Hg).

■ Normal heart rate is 120 to 160 beats per minute, except for increases during normal hyperactivity.

■ Normal temperature is 36.4°C (97.5°F) to 37.2°C (99°F).

■ Airway, APGAR, ID tags.

■ Promote bonding.

■ Promote breast feeding.

■ Monitor stools.

■ A formula-fed baby has one to two stools per day.

■ A breast-fed baby has 6 to 10 loose stools per day or one stool every few days.

■ Voiding pattern: wet diaper 6 to 8 times per day.

■ Umbilical cord care: clean cord with alcohol at each diaper change. Cord will fall off in 7 to 14 days.

■ Infants will receive antibiotics instilled in eyes, phytonadione (AquaMEPHYTON): vitamin K for clotting; hepatitis B vaccine.

■ PKU (after first feeding), Rh, Coombs' testing.

POINT TO PONDER

Baby should produce meconium (greenish-black) in 24 hours. Transitional stools are thin and brown to green and loose; they then become soft, yellow stool.

Cesarean Section

■ Reasons for failure to progress in labor can include fetal distress, prolapsed cord, cephalopelvic disproportion, malpresentation, abruptio placenta, placenta previa, herpes, and breech presentation.

Postdelivery Nursing Management Considerations

■ Encourage maternal/paternal bonding.

■ Taking-in phase: 1 to 2 days after delivery; dependent, passive; review labor.

■ Taking-hold phase: 2 to 4 days; dependent–independent.

■ Letting-go phase: after 4 days; family reorganization/autonomy and independence.

■ Postpartum depression:
Normal: letdown is mild and transient.
Depression/blues appears 2 to 3 days postpartum and lasts about 2 weeks.

PART IV

▶ Pharmacology

acetaminophen   *Tylenol, Liquiprim, Panadol, Anacin-3*

Use
Fever reduction, relief of mild-to-moderate pain

Adverse Reactions
Hepatotoxicity; acute renal failure

Client Education Information
Should avoid over-the-counter (OTC) preparations that also contain acetaminophen.

Consuming high-carbohydrate meals while taking medication at mealtime may inhibit absorption.

Consumption of alcohol while taking acetaminophen can make clients more prone to hepatotoxicity.

albuterol   *Ventolin, Proventil (via inhaler)*

POINT TO PONDER

Teach client to shake all inhalers thoroughly, exhale, then inhale with lips around mouthpiece.

Use
Relieves bronchospasm of acute/chronic asthma and bronchitis

Adverse Reactions
As a sympathomimetic, it stimulates the cardiovascular system.

Client Education Information
Side effects can lead to tremors and nausea/vomiting.

If multiple inhalation medications are used, the client should use albuterol first, followed by steroids.

Clients should wait at least 5 minutes between administration of these inhalation medications.

allopurinol   *Zyloprim*

Use
Antigout

Adverse Reactions
Agranulocytosis, aplastic anemia, bone marrow depression

Client Education Information
The client should be encouraged to increase fluid intake to 2500 to 3000 mL per day (unless contraindicated).

Client should wear UV-protected sunglasses because exposure to ultraviolet light may cause cataracts.

High-purine foods such as organ meats, dried peas, beans, asparagus, cauliflower, salmon, and sardines should be limited.

Colchicine is used for *acute* episodes of gout.

Mylanta

aluminum hydroxide, magnesium hydroxide, and simethicone

Use
Antacid

Adverse Reactions
Diarrhea, constipation

Client Education Information
Teach clients to avoid taking antacids at the same time as they take other medications because it may hinder absorption of the other medications.

Aluminum-based preparations will produce constipation, while magnesium-based preparations will produce diarrhea in many clients.

Fungizone

amphotericin B

Use
Systemic antifungal used for fatal systemic mycotic infections, including cryptococcosis

Adverse Reactions
Nephrotoxicity

POINT TO PONDER

Never mix amphotericin B with saline.

Client Education Information
Advise clients taking intravenous forms of preparation to flush all lines with D_5W.

The intravenous administration should be delivered slowly over 6 hours.

Sunlight will affect the stability, so the medication should be protected from light during administration.

Blood tests will be required to monitor blood urea nitrogen (BUN).

Omnipen

ampicillin

Use
Antibiotic, anti-infective

Adverse Reactions
Anaphylactic reaction, pseudomembranous colitis

Client Education Information
Teach client to take the medication on an empty stomach.

Pharmacology

amoxicillin   *Amoxil*

Use
Antibiotic

Adverse Reactions
Agranulocytosis, anaphylaxis

Client Education Information
This medication may be given with food.

Advise the client that an ampicillin-specific rash may *not* be due to hypersensitivity, and it may start immediately after the drug is started.

If clients experience an itching rash after a few days, they may have developed a hypersensitivity.

---

angiotensin-converting enzyme (ACE inhibitors)   *captopril/Capoten, enalapril/Vasotec, lisinopril/Prinavil, Zestril*

Use
Antihypertensive

Adverse Reactions
Agranulocytosis; angioedema—especially swelling of the glottis/larynx; hyperkalemia

Client Education Information
Advise clients to avoid using any potassium-containing salt substitutes.

Clients should be monitored for episodes of hypotension.

The medication should be administered 1 hour before meals (give captopril on an empty stomach).

---

aspirin   *Bayer, Ecotrin*

Use
Antipyretic, mild-to-moderate pain relief, anti-inflammatory, low dose to prevent platelet aggregation

Adverse Reactions
(GI) bleeding, anaphylactic shock, tinnitus, impaired renal function

Client Education Information
Have the client take the medication with food or milk.

Never crush the enteric-coated aspirin.

Report ringing in the ears, as this is associated with chronic overdose.

POINTS TO PONDER

Aspirin is associated with Reye's syndrome. Do not give to children or teenagers, especially those with varicella.

Stop all aspirin intake at least 1 week prior to surgery to reduce chances of uncontrolled bleeding.

Atropisol, Isopto Atropine   **atropine**

Use

Anticholinergic; used for sinus bradycardia; also used preoperatively to decrease secretions; ophthalmic use to cause mydriasis (dilated pupil) prior to refraction

Adverse Reactions

Ventricular tachycardia, ventricular fibrillation, paralytic ileus; contraindicated with glaucoma

Client Education Information

Inform the client that the medication may cause urinary retention.

Elderly clients may become confused.

Infants and small children may develop hyperpyrexia.

When taking this medication, frequent mouth care should be administered.

This medication is used to treat mushroom poisoning.

Lioresal   **baclofen**

Use

Skeletal muscle relaxant; used in multiple sclerosis

Adverse Reactions

Mental confusion, hallucinations, especially in the elderly; adverse effects resemble diseases drug is used to treat

Client Education Information

Diabetics should assess capillary blood sugars for increased gluocose levels.

The medication should be discontinued gradually.

---

pentobarbital/Nembutal, secobarbital/Seconal, phenobarbital/Luminal   **barbiturates**

Use

Antianxiety, sedative, anticonvulsant

Adverse Reactions

CNS depression, addiction

Client Education Information

These are controlled substances that should be evaluated with each prescription.

Should not be discontinued abruptly.

Children and the elderly may experience paradoxical excitement.

benzodiazepines

diazepam/Valium, chlordiazepoxide/Librium, oxazepam/Serax, triazolam/Halcion

Use
Antianxiety drugs (formerly called sedatives)

Adverse Reactions
Drowsiness, sluggishness, impaired motor coordination, confusion, disorientation

Client Education Information
These are controlled substances and need close monitoring.
Instruct client to refrain from alcohol consumption.
Psychological and physiological addiction are possible, so teach clients not to overmedicate.

benztropine mesylate

Cogentin

Use
Treatment of Parkinson's disease

Adverse Reactions
Sedation, drowsiness, irritability, constipation, dry mouth, paralytic ileus, atropine-like side effects

Client Education Information
Instruct client to take medication after meals.
Dosage may need to be decreased in warmer weather.

beta blockers

atenolol/Tenormin, metoprolol/Lopressor, nadolol/Corgard, propranolol/Inderal

Use
Management of hypertension; reduces heart rate; Inderal used for migraines

Adverse Reactions
Bronchospasm, especially in those with a history of asthma or bronchoconstrictive disease; bradycardia; may mask symptoms of hypoglycemia; decreased sexual function; impotence in men

Client Education Information
Teach client how to check pulse rate and to hold medication and notify health care provider if pulse is less than 60 per minute.

Diprosone, Diprolene, Celestone, Betacort, Valisone

Use
Long-acting glucocorticoid with strong anti-inflammatory, immunosuppressive actions; used topically for inflammatory dermatologic disorders; used systemically in pregnant women for prevention of respiratory distress syndrome in neonates

Adverse Reaction
Fluid retention; Cushing's syndrome

Client Education Information
When topical preparation is used, the client should watch skin for signs of irritation.

May cause weight gain when given systemically.

Tell client not to stop taking medication suddenly.

May be given to mothers 2 to 3 days prior to delivery.

---

nifedipine/Procardia, Adalat; verapamil/Calan, Isoptin; diltiazem/Cardizem

calcium channel blockers

Use
Used with vasospastic (Prinzmetal's) angina; verapamil is used with supraventricular tachyarrhythmias

Adverse Reactions
Headache, dizziness, flushing, weakness, hypotension, nausea, edema, arrhythmias

Client Education Information
Have client learn how to take pulse.

Never stop this medication abruptly.

Sinemet

carbidopa–levodopa

Use
Treatment of Parkinson's disease

Adverse Reactions
Depression with suicidal tendencies, agranulocytosis, neuroleptic malignant syndrome

Client Education Information
Inform clients that they may develop involuntary facial movements and to notify physician if this occurs.

Should be used with caution in clients with glaucoma.

POINT TO PONDER

"On–off" syndrome occurs as a sudden recurrence of symptoms as drug wears off.

Pharmacology

cephalosporins

cefazolin/Ancef, Kefzol; cephalothin/Keflin; cefoxitin/Mefoxin; cefuroxime/Zinacef, cephalexin/Keflex, cefaclor/Ceclor, cefadroxil/Duricef

Use
Broad-spectrum antibiotic

Adverse Reactions
Allergic reactions, anaphylaxis, skin rash, fever, urticaria, diarrhea, nausea, vomiting

Client Education Information
This medication should be used cautiously in persons sensitive to penicillin.
Teach client to complete course of therapy.
This medication may be taken with food.

cimetidine

Tagamet

Use
H_2 receptor antagonist; suppresses gastric acid secretion

Adverse Reactions
Gynecomastia, confusion (especially in elderly)

Client Education Information
Instruct client to take 1 hour before or 2 hours after eating.
Do not take medication with antacids.
Should not be used in older adults.

codeine sulfate

Use
Narcotic, moderate pain reliever, antitussive

Adverse Reactions
Respiratory depression, circulatory collapse, anaphylactic reaction, constipation

Client Education Information
Nausea is a common side effect.
Client should avoid drinking alcohol, including alcohol found in some OTC cough preparations.

desmopressin acetate

DDAVP

Use
Synthetic pituitary hormone; used for diabetes insipidus

Adverse Reactions
Can cause fluid volume overload

Client Education Information
This medication may be given parenterally or nasally.
When medication is used, client should expect that urine output will decrease and specific gravity of urine will increase.

Pharmacology

Lanoxin   **digoxin**

Use
Cardiac glycoside used in congestive heart failure (CHF), atrial fibrillation

Adverse Reactions
Bradycardia, heart block, visual disturbances, GI upset

Client Education Information
Should take potassium replacement as toxicity potential increases with low serum potassium level.
Teach client to hold medication if heart rate is lower than 60 (therapeutic range, 0.8–2.0 ng/mL; toxic, above 2.0 ng/mL).

Benadryl hydrochloride   **diphenhydramine**

Use
Antihistamine used for allergic reactions, hay fever, cough; potent antiemetic

Adverse Reactions
Cardiovascular collapse, hypersensitivity

Client Education Information
Inform client that medication causes drowsiness, sedation, and dry mouth.
May be used during episodes of colds for its drying effect.
Do not drive when using.
When given parenterally, it will be given IM only.

Antabuse   **disulfiram**

Use
Deters alcohol ingestion

Adverse Reactions
Hypotension due to shock, arrhythmias, acute CHF, respiratory depression, convulsions, sudden death, psychoses

Client Education Information
Teach client not to ingest alcohol in any form, such as in cough medicines and foods, or in topical form, such as rubbing alcohol.

Colace   **docusate sodium**

Use
Stool softener

Adverse Reactions
(Rarely occur) abdominal cramps, diarrhea, nausea

Client Education Information
Instruct client to take with a glass of water to enhance effect.
Do not take along with mineral oil.

Pharmacology

epinephrine hydrochloride   *Adrenalin chloride*

Use
Potent sympathomimetic used in cardiac arrest, acute bronchospasm; strengthens myocardial contractions; ophthalmic preparations used in glaucoma; anaphylaxis

Adverse Reactions
Hypertension, myocardial infarction (MI), ventricular fibrillation, pulmonary edema, tremors

Client Education Information
When given by inhalation, client should rinse mouth after dose to avoid swallowing the drug.

▶ SAFETY TIP

Carefully aspirate syringe when giving SC (subcutaneously) or IM to prevent IV injection.

erythromycin   *Ilotycin, E-Mycin*

Use
Broad-spectrum antibacterial, similar in scope to penicillin, but used as a substitute in persons allergic to penicillin

Adverse Reactions
Hypersensitivity reactions—urticaria, fever, anaphylaxis, very irritating to the stomach; causes nausea, vomiting, abdominal cramps, anorexia

Client Education information
Encourage client to take with food if GI symptoms appear.
When ophthalmic preparation is used, teach client to avoid touching tube or dropper to eye and to wash hands thoroughly prior to administering.

estrogen replacement therapy   *Premarin, Estrace, Estratab, Ogen*

Use
Alleviates vasomotor symptoms associated with menopause; used postmenopause to lessen risk of osteoporosis and heart disease

Adverse Reactions
Fluid retention, breakthrough bleeding, increased risk of endometrial cancer, thromboembolic disease

Client Education Information
Women who have a uterus should cycle estrogen with progesterone; those without should take estrogen only. Women on estrogen replacement therapy should have annual gynecologic exams with Pap smear, as well as mammograms.

Prozac   **fluoxetine hydrochloride**

Use
Selective serotonin-reuptake inhibitor/antidepressant

Adverse Reactions
May interact with tryptophan, monoamine oxidase (MAO) inhibitors; increases the half-life of diazepam (Valium), nausea

Client Education Information
Teach client and family to assess for suicidal ideation.

Have client monitor weight.

Encourage client to take dose in A.M. to prevent insomnia.

Garamycin, Garamycin Ophthalmic   **gentamicin**

Use
Antibiotic

Adverse Reactions
Ototoxic, can produce hearing loss; nephrotoxic

Client Education Information
Instruct client to have frequent hearing assessments.

Cortisone, Deltasone, Decadron, Prednisone   **glucocorticoids**

Use
Potent anti-inflammatories; suppression of the immune system

Adverse Reactions
Hyperlipidemia, osteoporosis, weight gain, "moon face," mood swings, peptic and gastric ulcer, glaucoma, cataracts, hypertension and edema, hypokalemia, increased susceptibility to infection, poor wound healing

Client Education Information
Instruct client to take medication with food, antacids, or H_2 receptor antagonist.

Do not discontinue suddenly, taper dose.

Clients should avoid crowds and people with infections.

Diet should limit high-sodium foods.

Instruct client to report any infections, as glucocorticoids mask signs.

Robitussin, Guaituss   **guaifenesin**

Use
Expectorant

Adverse Reactions
Low incidence of side effects, GI upset, nausea, drowsiness

Client Education Information
Instruct client to drink extra fluids to assist in liquefying bronchial secretions.

When taken alone, this drug is *not* a cough suppressant; other drugs, such as codeine or dextromethorphan, may be used in combination with guaifenesin.

Pharmacology

haloperidol

Haldol

Use
Antipsychotic

Adverse Reactions
Tardive dyskinesia, neuroleptic syndrome, agranulocytosis, laryngospasm, respiratory depression

Client Education Information
Instruct client to not drink alcohol when taking this drug; do not mix liquid form with tea or coffee, as it will form a precipitate.

heparin (calcium)

Use
Anticoagulant; prevents thromboemboli

Adverse Reactions
Spontaneous bleeding

POINT TO PONDER

Antidote for heparin is protamine sulfate 1%.

Client Education Information
PTT (partial thromboplastin time), APTT (activated partial thromboplastin time) should be 1.5 to 2.5 times normal.
Teach bleeding precautions, including using soft toothbrush, no razors for shaving, no aspirin, no nonsteroidal anti-inflammatory drugs (NSAIDs).
This medication is given by SC/IV only.
Instruct clients that SC injections are into fat and that the nurse does not aspirate or rub; rotate sites.
Intravenous medication is preferably given via an infusion pump.

hepatitis B vaccine (recombinant)

Recombivax HB

Use
Promotes active immunity in individuals at high risk for exposure to the hepatitis B virus.

Adverse Reactions
Local swelling at injection site, fever, malaise, headache, hypersensitivity reaction

Client Education Information
Adults receive a series of three injections on days 1, 30, and 180. Children receive vaccine at birth, 1 month, and 6 months.

hydralazine

Apresoline

Use
Reduces blood pressure in moderate-to-severe hypertension

Adverse Reactions
Shock, agranulocytosis, arrhythmias

Client Education Information
Advise client to change position slowly to avoid postural hypotension; some persons experience palpitations after first dose.
Teach client to monitor weight and check for edema.

hydroxyzine hydrochloride/Atarax; hydroxyzine pamoate/Vistaril

hydroxyzine

Use
Antihistamine, antipruritic; antiemetic

Adverse Reactions
Drowsiness, dry mouth

Client Education Information
Client should have frequent mouth care.

Humulin, Novolin, Velosulin

insulin

Use
Antidiabetic, type I diabetes

Adverse Reactions
Hypoglycemic reaction, anaphylaxis

Client Education Information
Teach client signs and symptoms of hypoglycemia.

Instruct on assessing blood sugar frequently and self-injection.

Regular insulin may be mixed with other insulins (draw up regular first).

Teach client to rotate injection sites to prevent lipodystrophy.

Instruct client to not rub injection site.

---

ipecac syrup

Use
Emetic; induces vomiting

Adverse Reactions
Diarrhea; if drug is absorbed, persistent vomiting, cardiomyopathy, cardiotoxicity, cardiac arrhythmias, hypotension

Client Education Information
Make sure client does not confuse with ipecac fluid extract, which is 14 times stronger and will cause death if given at the same dose.

Client should consume with warm water, *not* milk or carbonated beverages.

May repeat in 20 to 30 minutes; if no vomiting occurs, contact physician immediately.

INH

isoniazid

Use
Treatment of tuberculosis (TB)

Adverse Reactions
Paresthesias, peripheral neuropathy, agranulocytosis, aplastic anemia

Client Education Information
Instruct client to take on an empty stomach and to take vitamin B_6 supplements often, as drug interferes with absorption of B_6.

May produce false positives with Clinitest.

Pharmacology

ketoconazole

Nizoral

Use
Antifungal, for severe systemic fungal infections

Adverse Reactions
Nausea, vomiting, acute hypoadrenalism, anaphylaxis, angioedema, skin rash, urticaria

Client Education Information
Nausea and vomiting may occur frequently.
Client should avoid alcohol.

lactulose

Cephulac, Chronulac

Use
Treatment of portal-systemic encephalopathy; unlabeled use for chronic constipation and the restoration of regular bowel habits posthemorrhoidectomy

Adverse Reactions
Diarrhea is a sign of overdosage

Client Education Information
Inform client that the drug takes 2 to 3 days to produce soft stools; promote fluid intake.

levodopa

L-dopa, Laradopa, Dopar

Use
Treatment of Parkinson's disease

Adverse Reactions
Involuntary movements (chorea), ataxia, confusion, agitation, anxiety, insomnia, psychosis and delusions, depression; blepharospasm, anorexia, nausea, vomiting, dry mouth, dysphagia

Client Education Information
Diabetic clients may experience changes in blood sugar.
Clients may become lightheaded or dizzy because of orthostatic hypotension (caution them to arise from bed slowly).
May experience some abnormal movements such as grimacing, tongue protrusion, bobbing of head, jerky arm movements, spasmodic winking.
Instruct client to report these immediately, as they reprsent signs of overdose.

levothyroxine

Levothroid, Synthroid

Use
Synthetic thyroid hormone for thyroid replacement

Adverse Reactions
Irritability, insomnia, tremors, palpitations, tachycardia, hypertension, GI upset, nausea, diarrhea, change in appetite, menstrual irregularities

Client Education Information
Instruct client to take a single dose prior to breakfast, as food interferes with absorption.
Instruct client not to stop drug suddenly.

Eskalith, Lithobid, Lithotabs

lithium

Use
Mixed bipolar disorder

Adverse Reactions
Peripheral circulatory collapse, leukocytosis, nephrogenic diabetes insipidus, hypothyroidism

Client Education Information
Client needs frequent blood monitoring for therapeutic level (0.6 to 1.5 mEq/L).

Client should monitor weight daily and report fluid gains and losses.

Client should drink 2 to 3 liters of fluid a day and replace 6 to 10 grams of sodium a day in hot weather.

Instruct client regarding the side effects, which include vomiting, diarrhea, lack of coordination, muscular weakness, and slurred speech.

Side effects progress when levels exceed 2.0 mEq/L, and include ataxia, blurred vision, tinnitus, muscle twitching, tremors, and a large output of dilute urine.

---

bumetadine/Bumex, ethacrynic acid/Edecrin, furosemide/Lasix

loop diuretics

Use
Potent diuretics that inhibit reabsorption along the ascending loop of Henle.

Adverse Reactions
Postural hypotension, hypokalemia, ototoxicity, aplastic anemia, agranulocytosis

Client Education Information
Encourage client to eat foods high in potassium.

Client may need to take potassium supplements as well.

Avoid taking medication at bedtime to prevent nocturia.

Teach client to report any hearing changes.

Ativan

lorazepam

Use
Antianxiety

Adverse Reactions
Addiction, sedation

Client Education Information
Client should not drive; should avoid alcohol.

lovastatin *Mevacor*

Use
Antilipemic (lowers serum lipids)

Adverse Reactions
Increases serum transaminase, creatine kinase

Client Education Information
This medication may cause GI disturbances.

Clients who have a history of alcohol use or liver disease should be advised to abstain.

Take with meals.

Have client return for liver function tests every 1 to 2 months during first year of therapy.

Client should report muscle aches and pains.

---

magaldrate *Riopan*

Use
Antacid

Adverse Reactions
Can cause diarrhea or constipation

Client Education Information
Caution clients to not take this medication with other medications, as it may interfere with the absorption of them.

This antacid is low in sodium and good for sodium restricted clients.

---

magnesium sulfate *Epsom salt*

Use
Taken orally, it acts as a laxative by osmotic retention of fluid; administered parenterally, it acts as a CNS depressant of smooth, skeletal, and cardiac muscle.

Parenterally, it is used to treat seizures associated with toxemia of pregnancy.

Adverse Reactions
Complete heart block, circulatory collapse, respiratory paralysis

Client Education Information
Advise client to report side effects.

Oral medication will taste bitter and salty and is best taken in morning or afternoon to minimize laxative effect.

When given IV, constant observation of blood pressure, pulse, and respirations is required.

Normal plasma levels are 1.8 to 3.0 mEq/L; levels in excess of 4.0 mEq/L are reflected in depressed deep tendon reflexes; more than 25 mEq/L results in cardiac arrest. Early signs of toxicity are a sense of warmth and muscle weakness.

Pharmacology

Osmitrol   **mannitol**

Use
Osmotic diuretic; used with increased intracranial pressure

Adverse Reactions
Hyponatremia, dehydration, extravasation when injected into tissues

Client Education Information
Client will require close monitoring of intake and output.
When given IV, maintain urine output 30 to 50 mL/hr by adjusting fluid infusion rate; crystallizes easily.

Reglan   **metoclopramide**

Use
Cholinergic GI agent, used to accelerate gastric emptying; used to treat gastric stasis and nausea and vomiting resulting from chemotherapy.

Adverse Reactions
Fatigue, restlessness, extrapyramidal symptoms, diarrhea, hypertensive crisis

Client Education Information
Client should be instructed to take this medication 30 minutes prior to meals and bedtime.
Instruct client to report rigidity, tremors, or facial grimacing.

Ritalin   **methylphenidate hyrdochloride**

Use
CNS stimulant; used in hyperkinetic syndromes and with attention deficit disorder

Adverse Reactions
Nervousness, insomnia, hepatotoxicity, exfoliative dermatitis

Client Education Information
Children should have baseline height and weight to monitor for loss of appetite.
Instruct client/parent to take/administer medication 30 to 45 minutes prior to meals.

Demerol   **meperidine hydrochloride**

Use
Synthetic narcotic, similar to morphine, for moderate-to-severe pain, used in obstetric anesthesia

Adverse Reactions
Respiratory depression, cardiovascular collapse, cardiac arrest

Client Education Information
Client may experience dizziness, nausea, vomiting, and faintness.
Teach client to abstain from alcohol while taking this medication.

Pharmacology

metronidazole	*Flagyl*

Use

Antitrichomonal (for *Trichomonas*) and amebicide for *Giardia lamblia* and *Entamoeba histolytica*)

Adverse Reactions

Nausea, overgrowth of *Candida*, CNS changes (including seizures, peripheral neuropathy), sodium retention

Client Education Information

Advise clients that they cannot drink alcohol when taking this medication, as it will cause an acute psychotic reaction.

monamine oxidase (MAO) inhibitors	*Marplan, Nardil, Parnate*

Use

Antidepressant

Adverse Reactions

Drowsiness, dry mouth, orthostatic hypotension, blurred vision, dysuria; constipation

Client Education Information

Clients taking MAO inhibitors must maintain strict dietary avoidance of foods containing tyramine, such as aged cheese, avocados, red wine, and beer, as they can precipitate a hypertensive crisis.

morphine

Use

Narcotic analgesic for severe pain, opiate

Adverse Reactions

Respiratory depression, cardiovascular collapse, cardiac arrest, anaphylaxis, high abuse potential

Client Education Information

Encourage family members to assess respiratory status prior to dose.

This medication may be given with an antiemetic to reduce nausea/vomiting.

For oncology pain, develop a regular dosing schedule.

Given for myocardial infarction (MI) pain.

Teach clients not to take if they have pancreatic/biliary (gallbladder pain), as it causes spasm of the sphincter of Oddi. Contraindicated in conditions such as cholecystitis or pancreatitis.

Narcan   naloxone hydrochloride

Use

In acute opiate overdose, to reverse the effect of narcotics; give IV only

Adverse Reactions

Nausea, vomiting, sweating, tremors, tachycardia

Client Education Information

This medication is given for overdose.

Respiratory assessment is critical to assess respiratory status.

Narcan may wear off before opiate; thus, respiration rate may fall again.

Isosorbide dinitrate/Isordil, nitroglycerin   nitrates

Use

Relaxes smooth muscle, thus dilating arteries

Adverse Reactions

Potent vasodilation, hypotension, flushing, headache

Client Education Information

Teach client to rotate sites with topical preparations; avoid hairy areas.

Caregiver should avoid getting topical ointment on hands.

Inform clients that sublingual tablets should burn slightly under the tongue.

If no relief is obtained, then repeat after 5 minutes and again in another 5 minutes if necessary. If no relief is obtained after three tablets, advise client to seek medical attention.

Teach client to not move medication out of original container into light.

Replace unopened bottle every 6 months.

---

naproxen/Naprosyn, Aleve; ibuprofen/Advil, Motrin   NSAIDs

Use

For pain relief; relief of inflammation; antipyretic

Adverse Reactions

Aplastic anemia, toxic hepatitis, anaphylaxis

Client Education Information

Advise clients to take with food.

They should not take this medication if they have an allergy to aspirin.

Clients should avoid high-sodium foods as this medication may cause water retention.

Mycostatin   nystatin

Use

Antifungal

Adverse Reactions

Usually mild, nausea, vomiting, epigastric distress

Client Education Information

This medication is given PO for oral candidiasis.

Oral liquid ordered as a "swish and spit" or "swish and swallow" when treating thrush.

Teach clients to remove dentures prior to rinsing mouth.

Pharmacology

oxycodone hydrochloride

Percocet, Percodan, Roxicet

Use
Narcotic/pain reliever

Adverse Reactions
Respiratory depression/hepatotoxicity

Client Education Information
Teach client that Percocet contains acetaminophen; Percodan contains aspirin and can cause gastric irritation and constipation.
Client should take this medication with food.

♀ POINT TO PONDER

Assess for aspirin allergy with Percodan; acetaminophen allergy with Percocet.

pancrelipase

Pancrease, Viokase

Use
Pancreatic enzyme used in malabsorption due to cystic fibrosis and other exocrine pancreatic insufficiency

Adverse Reactions
Nausea, vomiting, anorexia, diarrhea

Client Education Information
Inform client that this medication should not be crushed (enteric tablets).
Teach client/family member to take/give medication with meals.
Powdered form sprinkled on food (for children).

penicillin

penicillin VK/Pen Vee K; penicillin G/Pentids

Use
Antibiotic

Adverse Reactions
Anaphylaxis; rash, pruritus

Client Education Information
Teach client to finish prescription; take around the clock.
(IM preparation should be given into deep muscle, aspirate carefully to avoid possible accidental IV administration.)

phenothiazines

chlorpromazine/Thorazine, prochlorperazine/Compazine, thioridazine/Mellaril

Use
Antipsychotic; Compazine is used for its antiemetic effect

Adverse Reactions
Extrapyramidal side effects include pseudoparkinsonism (rigidity), tremors, pill rolling; acute dystonia (abnormal posturing); akathisia (inability to sit still); tardive dyskinesia (involuntary, rhythmic, bizarre movements of face, jaw, mouth, and tongue)

Client Education Information
Teach client to rise slowly to avoid orthostatic hypotension; males may avoid medication due to impotence.
Client may experience a feeling of being cold.
Teach client/family about signs and symptoms of CNS depression.

Pharmacology

Dilantin   **phenytoin**

Use
Antiseizure; antiarrhythmic

Adverse Reactions
Aplastic anemia, agranulocytosis, cardiovascular collapse

Client Education Information
Client should be taught how to provide meticulous mouth care, as drug can cause hyperplasia of gums.
Assess for evidence of infiltration as it causes severe soft tissue irritation.

Minipress   **prazosin**

Use
alpha-adrenergic blocker to treat hypertension

Adverse Reactions
Hypotension, dizziness, palpitations, allergic reactions.

Client Education Information
Client may develop severe hypotension after the first dose.

Propyl-Thracil   **propylthiouracil (PTU)**

Use
Synthetic antithyroid hormone; used in hyperthyroidism

Adverse Reactions
Agranulocytosis, hypothyroidism

Client Education Information
Teach client that excess dosage signs include mental depression, muscle twitching (when pricked), hard and nonpitting edema, and an intolerance to cold.

Sudafed   **pseudoephedrine hydrochloride**

Use
Decongestant (α- and β-adrenergic agonist)

Adverse Reactions
Tremors, tachycardia, nervousness, sleeplessness, anorexia, dry mouth, nausea/vomiting

Client Education Information
Clients with a history of hypertension should not use.
Client should avoid taking near bedtime to avoid sleeplessness.
Teach client to avoid using other OTC medications that might contain other ephedrine-like drugs.

Pharmacology

psyllium   *Metamucil*

Use
GI bulking agent, laxative

Adverse Reaction
Diarrhea, nausea, vomiting, abdominal cramps

Client Education Information
Encourage fluid intake.
May be given via NG tube with tube feedings to provide bulk and lessen diarrhea.

quinidine gluconate   *Quinaglute*

Use
Antiarrhythmic

Adverse Reactions
Heart block, widened QRS, ventricular fibrillation/ventricular flutter, acute hemolytic anemia, agranulocytosis, respiratory depression, cinchonism (characterized by tinnitus, decreased auditory acuity, dizziness, vertigo, and headache). (Quinidine comes from the bark of the cinchona tree.)

Client Education Information
Teach client not to eat excessive amounts of fruits and vegetables (ie, vegetarian diet).
(Therapeutic level, 2 to 5 mg/L; levels of 8 mg/L or more are considered toxic.)

ranitidine   *Zantac*

Use
H_2 receptor antagonist suppresses gastric acid secretion

Adverse Reactions
Less side effects than Tagamet

Client Education Information
Smoking decreases effect; may be given with food; some antacids decrease absorption (ie, Mylanta II).

rifampin   *Rifadin, Rimactane*

Use
Treatment of TB

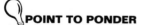
POINT TO PONDER

Rifampin may impart a harmless red-orange color to urine, feces, sputum, sweat, and tears; soft contact lenses may be permanently stained.

Adverse Reactions
Hepatorenal syndrome; acute renal failure

Client Education Information
Client should take medication on an empty stomach.
Instruct client to leave desiccant (the packet that absorbs moisture) in bottle, as moisture renders the drug unstable.
Clients using oral contraceptives should use another method of birth control, as rifampin decreases the effectiveness of oral contraceptives.

Use
Antacid; used as home remedy for heartburn, indigestion; also as a paste for minor skin irritations; used IV to correct metabolic acidosis

Adverse Reactions
Metabolic alkalosis, sodium overload, IV may cause intracranial hemorrhage

Client Education Information
Teach client side effects of long-term use, including anorexia, hypercalcemia, renal and ureteral calculi, and metabolic alkalosis.

Over-the-counter (OTC) preparations include Alka-Seltzer, Bromo-Seltzer, and Gaviscon.

Kayexalate

Use
Resin exchange agent for hyperkalemia (used in renal failure)

Adverse Reactions
Constipation, fecal impaction, anorexia, gastric irritation, nausea, vomiting, diarrhea

Client Education Information
This medication is administered via retention enema. Client should retain for 30 to 60 minutes.

Flush bowel with one to two quarts of nonsodium solution.

Client may experience hypokalemia.

Aldactone

Use
Potassium-sparing diuretic

Adverse Reactions
Fluid and electrolyte imbalances

Client Education Information
Inform males that use may create gynecomastia (growth of breasts).

Assess for hyperkalemia/hyponatremia.

Aldactazide

Use
Potassium-sparing diuretic and thiazide diuretic together

Adverse Reactions
Hyperkalemia, volume depletion

Client Education Information
Inform client to avoid salt substitutes containing potassium.

Pharmacology

sucralfate	*Carafate*

Use
Antiulcer; binds with gastric acid to form barriers

Adverse Reactions
Nausea, gastric discomfort, constipation, diarrhea

Client Education Information
Client should take this medication before meals and alone, as it may bind to other medications.

💡**POINT TO PONDER**

Do not crush tablet; for use in NG/G/J tubes, place tablet in small amount of water and it will quickly dissolve.

sulfonamides	*sulfamethoxazole/Gantanol; sulfisoxazole/Gantrisin*

Use
Anti-infective, used widely for urinary tract infections (UTIs), otitis media, vaginal infections, eye infections

Adverse Reactions
Anaphylaxis, allergic reactions, aplastic anemia, agranulocytosis, fever, chills

Client Education Information
Encourage client to increase fluid intake to prevent crystals from forming in kidney.
Women taking oral contraceptives should use another method of birth control.
Client must avoid exposure to sun (use sunscreen, even in cool/cold weather).

terbutaline sulfate	*Brethine, Brethaire*

Use
β-Adrenergic agonist; opens bronchial tree; also used to stop premature labor

Adverse Reactions
Tremor, lightheadedness, tachycardia, palpitations

Client Education Information
Instruct client not to use any other OTC inhaler.

theophylline	*Theo-Dur, Slo-Bid, Slo-Phyllin*

Use
Bronchodilator

Adverse Reactions
Tremors, irritability, insomnia, drug-induced seizures, circulatory failure, respiratory arrest

Client Education Information
Inform clients that granules may be mixed with food.
(Proper dosing schedule is important for maximum effect; limit caffeine to reduce possible adverse effects. Therapeutic level, 10 to 20 μg/mL; levels above 20 μg/mL are associated with toxicity.)

Pharmacology

chlorothiazide/Diuril, hydrochlorothiazide/Hydrodiuril   **thiazides**

Use
Diuretic

Adverse Reactions
Paresthesias, lightheadedness, orthostatic hypotension, agranulocytosis, aplastic anemia

Client Education Information
Client with diabetes should be taught that drug may cause loss of glycemic control.
Client should take medication early in the day to prevent nocturia.
Encourage foods high in potassium to replace kidney losses.

Mellaril   **thioridazine hydrochloride**

Use
Antipsychotic

Adverse Reactions
Paralytic ileus; may cause extrapyramidal syndrome

Client Education Information
Inform client the medication may cause urinary retention, constipation, and color urine pink/brown.

Imipramine hydrochloride/Tofranil, amitriptyline/Elavil,   **tricyclic antidepressants**
doxepin/Sinequan, nortriptyline/ Pamelor

Use
Treatment of endogenous depression; Tofranil (imipramine) is used to treat enuresis

Adverse Reactions
Parkinsonian effects, tardive dyskinesia, angioedema, agranulocytosis, urinary retention

Client Education Information
May take several weeks (2 to 4) for onset of action.

Artane   **trihexyphenidyl hydrochloride**

Use
Treatment of Parkinson's disease

Adverse Reactions
CNS stimulation—confusion, delirium; may cause urinary retention, constipation, dry mouth, blurred vision

Client Education Information
Client should take medication before or after meals.
Client should monitor bowel function.

Pharmacology

trimethoprim/sulfamethoxazole

Bactrim, Septra

Use
Anti-infective with sulfonamide; used in *Pneumocystis carinii* pneumonia, UTIs, bronchitis, otitis media in children

Adverse Reactions
Agranulocytosis, aplastic anemia, enterocolitis

Client Education Information
Teach client to drink extra fluids; avoid sunlight because of photosensitivity; assess for hyperglycemia.

vancomycin hydrochloride

Vancocin

Use
Used for life-threatening infections; orally, used with *Clostridium difficile* infections.

Adverse Reactions
Nephrotoxicity, ototoxicity, anaphylaxis, vascular collapse, hypotension with flushing of upper neck and face

Client Education Information
This medication is given IV over at least 1 hour; monitor IV site for infiltration (severe irritation and necrosis can occur); monitor peak and trough: peak is 20 to 30 mg/mL; trough < 15 mg/mL.
Client should report any ringing of the ears (tinnitus), hearing loss.
Cloudy, pink urine may be a sign of nephrotoxicity.

phytonadione (vitamin K1)

AquaMEPHYTON

Use
Clotting factor; antidote to counteract effect of Coumadin; used in newborns to prevent bleeding

Adverse Reactions
Anaphylaxis, bronchospasm, cardiac and respiratory arrest, death

Client Education Information
May be used in newborns, as it is not yet present in their GI tract.
Medication must be protected from light.

POINT TO PONDER

Vitamin K is used as the antidote to Coumadin overdose.

Pharmacology

Coumadin **warfarin**

Use
Anticoagulant/prevents blood clotting

Adverse Reactions
Spontaneous bleeding

Client Education Information
Client will have to have blood drawn to monitor prothrombin time (PT) (1.5 to 2.5 times control) (also described as international normalized ratio [INR]).

This medication is used for long-term anticoagulation.

Client should avoid foods high in vitamin K_1 as they may decrease effect (ie, cabbage, cauliflower, broccoli, asparagus, lettuce, spinach, or foods with caffeine).

Teach client bleeding precautions.

Advise client to discontinue at least 3 days prior to surgery.

Retrovir/AZT **zidovudine**

Use
Antiviral drug used in AIDS

Adverse Reactions
Anemia, granulocytopenia, myelosuppression

Client Education Information
Client may experience nausea and vomiting.

Medication does not cure HIV nor reduce transmission.

Used with HIV-positive persons who have CD4 counts less than or equal to 500/mm^3; used in combination with other antiviral drugs.

Pharmacology

PART V

▶ NCLEX-PN Review Books

- Comprehensive Review Books
- Question and Answer Books

When you approach studying for the NCLEX-PN CAT, you will find that there are a number of books available from which to select. These books are divided into two major categories: The "comprehensive review" book and the "question and answer"(Q & A) book. The comprehensive review book covers a variety of content areas and may include some test questions. The purpose of the comprehensive book is to assist you in brushing up on material you may have forgotten or may not have learned. The Q & A books are designed to test you in a multiple-choice format similar to that of the NCLEX-PN CAT exam. They usually provide test questions, along with the correct answers and rationales for why the answers are correct or incorrect. In addition to the books, you may see flash cards with questions and answers, computer disks with questions and answers, and even audio tapes to study by.

The purpose of this section is to provide you with an idea of the types of study guides available. This section will describe a number of books of the comprehensive review variety and in the Q & A category. The information will include the name of each book, the edition described, and the suggested retail price. The senior author will be noted, as well as the size of the book, the number of pages, and the ISBN number (this number may help you order the book from your bookstore if it is not available). This is followed by a description of the book, along with comments about the strengths and weaknesses of the work. In the upper left or right corner, a rating will be provided based on the rating system below. The ratings and comments about the book are provided by newly graduated practical nurses who have taken the NCLEX-PN CAT licensure examination.

Several words of caution are worth mentioning.

1. The retail prices of these books are as accurate as is known at the time of printing of this book and are subject to changes by the publisher, supplier, and bookstore, so use this as a guide only.

2. Every attempt to use the most recent edition of the books has been made, but new editions are constantly being published. This could affect the price, size, and even organization of the books as described, and whether or not they contain practice disks.

3. Sometimes a book may be reprinted with a different publisher or even a different author. If you are not able to find a specific review book, then speak with the bookstore manager.

The rating system for the books includes the following:

RATING	DESCRIPTOR
A+	The best used; none better
A	Excellent for review
A–	Very good for review
B+	Good for review
B	Good for review, but not strong
B–	Good for review, OK at times
C+	Fair, not completely satisfied
C	Fair for review
C–	Fair; many are better/more relevant
D	Not appropriate for review

The reviewer ratings and comments were based on a number of variables, including the readability of the book (understandability); format of the content being presented; the amount of information presented (the length and size does not necessarily make for a better book); the size of the sections in the book; the number of questions in the book; the quality of the questions; the quality of the rationales for correct and incorrect responses (and whether they are present); the size of the type of the book; the aesthetic appearance of the contents; and the paper used for printing the book. These ratings are related to the effectiveness and suitability of use for preparing for the NCLEX-PN CAT. When more than one book received the same rating, they are listed alphabetically by title.

The ratings and reviewer comments are based on informal surveys and critiques by graduate nurses from several nursing programs. The comments and overall ratings represent a compilation of opinions, and it should be noted that there was often a wide range of opinions about a particular item.

The rating was based on graduate nurses' opinions of the books as they relate to preparing exclusively for the NCLEX-PN CAT, and not to content accuracy. These books may have additional use during nursing programs for course work, but the ratings are not meant to reflect this.

Point to Ponder

The role of the licensed practical/vocational nurse is evolving rapidly, and the information being tested on the NCLEX-PN is being constantly updated. The recent job performance study, combined with the role delineation survey performed by the National Council of State Boards of Nursing, Inc., necessitate the continuous updating of review books. We strongly encourage your participation in offering your opinion on various review books and rating of books. Ratings of additional books and materials can be performed only with your help. We request that you take some time and return the book review form in the front of the book with your comments and ratings.

To contribute your comments and reviews, simply fill out the form using the rating system above, and include information about you, as requested, so we can verify your participation. We hope to make this book a valuable tool and resource for you and your future colleagues who will take the NCLEX-PN CAT after you.

Disclaimer: No material in this Part, including the ratings, reflect the opinion or influence of the publisher or author. All errors and omissions will be gladly corrected if brought to the attention of the author through the publisher.

B+

Content Review for the NCLEX-PN CAT, 6/e $27.95

Smith, S.

Appleton & Lange, 509 pages, 8 1/2" × 11", 1997, ISBN 0-8385-1516-9

Description: This book includes fourteen chapters. The first chapter describes ways to prepare for the NCLEX-PN examination, the testing procedure, and information about the test plan. Other chapters include information about nursing care throughout the life span, pharmacology, nutrition, and laboratory/diagnostic tests. A separate chapter addressing general nursing concepts includes items such as common procedures, recording/charting, communication skills, pre- and postoperative care, and physiologic information. Seven chapters are devoted to specialty areas, including medical–surgical nursing, oncologic nursing, emergency nursing, geriatric nursing, mental health nursing, maternity nursing, and pediatric nursing. A systems approach is used to organize the information within the medical–surgical and pediatric areas. Legal issues are discussed in a separate chapter. The final chapter includes two comprehensive tests; the rationales for correct and some incorrect responses are included. Questions are organized in a single-item, stand-alone format. A computer practice disk with 100 questions is supplied.

Comments

Strengths: Good content overview.
Strong review of fundamentals.
Print easy to read.

Weaknesses: Needs more practice questions.
Questions at the end of sections would be helpful.

B+

Mosby's Comprehensive Review of Practical Nursing, 11/e $28.95

Yannes-Eyles, M.

Mosby, 510 pages, 8 1/2" × 11", 1994, ISBN 0-8016-7006-3

Description: This book is organized into twelve chapters. The first section of the book describes the way to prepare for the NCLEX-PN examination. Other sections include anatomy and physiology, pharmacology, nursing process and basic practice, and current trends in nursing in North America. Specialty areas are divided into medical–surgical nursing, mental health nursing, obstetric nursing, pediatric nursing, gerontologic nursing, and emergency nursing. Review examinations are at the end of each chapter, and the correct answers, rationales for correct and incorrect answers, level of difficulty, nursing process category, and category of client needs are included at the end of the book. Information presented in the specialty chapters is organized in a modified systems approach format. Appendices contain various tables and charts for study. The final part of the book includes two comprehensive examinations, along with the correct answers, brief rationales for the correct and incorrect answers, level of difficulty, nursing process, and category of client needs. A computer practice disk with 100 questions is supplied.

Comments

Strengths: In-depth review of specific areas.
Good organization of material.
Excellent rationales to questions.

Weaknesses: Needs more test-taking information.
Needs to be more board specific.
Answers and rationales are hard to find.

NCLEX-PN New Study Guide for Practical Nursing $24.95

B+

Zerwekh, J. & Claborn, J.

Nursing Education Consultants, 474 pages, 8 1/2" × 11", 1992, ISBN 0-9628210-1-2

Description: This book contains twenty-two chapters. The first chapter focuses on test-taking strategies and principles of communication. Other chapters discuss growth and development; general nursing care concepts (including legal issues, pre- and postoperative care, and nutrition); and the concept of homeostasis. One chapter is devoted to pharmacology, one to psychiatric nursing, one to maternity nursing, one to care of the newborn, and another to trauma/emergency nursing. A modified systems approach is used for presentation of the sensory, endocrine, hematologic, respiratory, cardiac, gastrointestinal, hepatic, genitourinary, neurologic, and musculoskeletal systems. Anatomy and physiology information is provided within each section. NCLEX-PN information is supplied in one of the final sections. The last portion of this book is devoted to two comprehensive practice examinations. The questions in the examinations are a single-item format. Answers to the examinations include the correct response and rationales for correct and some incorrect answers. A computer practice disk is not supplied.

Comments

Strengths: Strong organization of information.
Nursing priorities are highlighted.
Good amount of information for review.

Weaknesses: Needs more practice questions.
Rationales lack depth for incorrect responses.

Saunders Review of Practical Nursing for NCLEX-PN, 2/e

$27.95

Matassarin-Jacobs, E.

W. B. Saunders, 476 pages, 8 1/2" × 11", 1992, ISBN 0-7216-3694-2

Description: This book contains ten sections of information. The first section describes the NCLEX-PN test format and how to prepare for the examination. The second section is devoted to test strategies and includes two practice tests, along with rationales for correct and incorrect answers, nursing process, category of client needs, and content area being tested. Other sections include the nursing process, pharmacology, maternity nursing, and care of the mental health client. The adult client section includes growth and development, reproductive disorders, and medical–surgical issues organized in a functional health pattern approach. The pediatric client section is organized in a similar fashion and also uses the functional health pattern approach as the organizing framework. The final portion includes two additional practice tests, along with rationales for correct and incorrect answers, nursing process, category of client needs, and content area being tested. The appendix includes additional NCLEX-PN information. A computer practice disk is not supplied.

Comments

Strengths: Content well organized.
            Good number of test questions.
            Rationales provide additional information.

Weaknesses: Not enough rationale information for incorrect responses.
            More illustrations would be helpful.

Davis's NCLEX-PN Review

$27.95

Beare, P.

F.A. Davis, 695 pages, 8 1/2" × 11", 1994, ISBN 0-8036-0671-0

Description: This book is divided into five parts. The first unit includes a description of how the test was developed and how to prepare for the examination. The second unit focuses on anatomy and physiology, legal issues, diagnostic studies, procedures, and growth and development. Unit three includes information about nutrition and pharmacology. The fourth unit focuses on clinical issues in pediatric nursing, older adult care, medical–surgical nursing, and maternity nursing areas. Unit four is organized in a systems approach format. Practice examinations are included at the end of each section in units three and four. The final unit consists of five integrated exams for practice. All examinations include the correct answers and rationales for correct answers and some incorrect answers; nursing process area (the term "Assessment" is used to refer to data collection items described in the NCLEX-PN examination), and category of client needs. The questions are organized in a case situation approach or single-item format. A computer practice disk with 450 questions is supplied.

Comments

Strengths: Good test-taking information.
Rationales for test questions.
Outline of diseases.

Weaknesses: Too much information included.
Needs more practice questions.
Needs more rationales for incorrect responses.

Barron's How to Prepare for the NCLEX-PN, 3/e $29.95

Curlin, V. & Allen, H.

Barron's, 474 pages, 8 1/2" × 11", 1995, ISBN 0-8120-8279-6

B⁻

Description: This book contains thirteen chapters, a mastery test, and several appendices. The introduction includes a discussion of the NCLEX-PN and how to prepare for the examination and a diagnostic test, which is followed by the correct answers with rationales for correct answers only, category of client needs, and nursing process category being tested. Chapters describe topics such as legal issues, basic nursing principles and procedures, basic sciences, public health, emergency and disaster nursing, and rehabilitation nursing. Specialty areas are presented in separate chapters and include nursing care of adult, pediatric, obstetric, gerontologic, oncologic, and mentally ill clients. Specialty area information is organized in a modified systems approach format. Appendices include abbreviation and immunization lists. A mastery examination using a case presentation method of testing is included. The correct answers, rationales for correct and some incorrect answers, category of client needs, and nursing process are also included. A computer practice disk with 500 questions is supplied.

Comments

Strengths: In-depth review of material.
Easy to read.
Rationales are good.

Weaknesses: Too much information provided.
Needs more review questions.

The Comprehensive NCLEX-PN Review, 3/e $29.95

Hoefler, P.

Meds, Inc., 348 pages, 8 1/2" × 11", 1997, ISBN 156533-023-4

B⁻

Description: This book contains five major units. The first unit describes test-taking strategies for the NCLEX-PN examination, including studying methods, strategies to answer questions, and ways to prepare for the test. Unit two includes information about medical–surgical issues presented in a modified systems approach format for areas such as the respiratory, cardiac, gastrointestinal, and genitourinary systems, and additional information about fluid and electrolytes, pre- and postoperative care, oncology nursing, and care of burns. The third unit describes major psychological problems such as anxiety, schizophrenia, personality disorders, and chemical dependency. Unit four covers maternal–child care information, including labor and delivery, pre- and postpartum care, and newborn care. The final unit presents material related to pediatric nursing, including acute illnesses, accidents, congenital abnormalities, and oncologic disorders. An appendix includes information about nutrition, calculations, and pharmacology. Nursing intervention sections are highlighted in gray blocks. No test questions are included in the book; however, a computer practice disk with 100 questions is supplied.

Comments

Strengths: Excellent testing tips.
                   Highlights intervention points.
                   Good tables with information.

Weaknesses: No questions are included in book.
                   Needs to reinforce learning through testing.

C+

American Nursing Review for NCLEX-PN, 2/e $27.95
Mourad, L.
Springhouse Corporation, 542 pages, 8 1/2" × 11", 1994, ISBN 0-87434-801-3

Description: This book contains five major parts. The first part includes a 63-item pretest, followed by the correct answers, rationales for correct and incorrect answers, category of client needs, and nursing process category for each question. The second section presents the test plan, understanding the examination, and strategies to improve success. Part three discusses general nursing principles and issues related to care including procedures such as changing a dressing or applying an ice pack. This section also includes information about legal issues, nutrition, and general physiologic principles. Part four is organized by specialty area, such as medical–surgical nursing, pediatric nursing, maternity nursing, oncologic nursing, and psychiatric nursing. The medical–surgical section is organized in a systems approach format, including the respiratory, cardiac, musculoskeletal, gastrointestinal, genitourinary, integumentary, and neurologic systems. Part five contains various appendices. The final section of this book contains a practice test, along with correct answers but not rationales for correct or incorrect responses. A computer practice disk with 150 questions is supplied.

Comments

Strengths: Review sections good for use during school.
                   In-depth assessment areas.
                   Tinted pages are easy to read.

Weaknesses: Information provided is too in-depth.
                   More questions would be helpful.
                   Review sections are not board specific.

The Complete Q & A Book for the NCLEX-PN $29.95

A⁻

Hoefler, P.

Meds, Inc., 384 pages, 8 ½" × 11", 1995, ISBN 1-56533-015-3

Description: This book contains an introduction, ten practice tests, and sections of correct answers to the tests. The introduction provides information about the NCLEX-PN, testing strategies, and a test analysis form. Each of the practice tests contains 100 questions of a single-item design organized in a comprehensive format. The index is organized to delineate each question using medical–surgical, psychiatric, pediatric, maternal–child, communication, pharmacologic, and test-taking strategies categories. The rationale sections repeat the questions in the examination followed by the correct answers and the rationales for correct and incorrect responses. Test-taking tips are included in rationale section. The questions in the examinations are designed in a single-item format. A computer practice disk with 100 questions is supplied.

Comments

Strengths: Good level of difficulty of questions.
             Good explanation of rationales for correct and incorrect responses.

Weaknesses: Print too small.

Review Questions for the NCLEX-PN, 3/e $21.95

B⁺

Smith, S.

Appleton & Lange, 226 pages, 8 1/2" × 11", 1997, ISBN 0-8385-8445-4

Description: This book contains seven parts. The first part describes the NCLEX-PN test plan design, the process of application, and obtaining examination results. The second part designs a review plan and presents test-taking strategies. Parts three and four include two comprehensive examinations and a self-assessment grid. Part five includes tests in specialty areas such as medical–surgical, maternity, pediatric, psychiatric, oncologic, nutrition, pharmacologic, geriatric, and legal areas. Parts six and seven include two comprehensive examinations, along with another self-assessment grid. Correct answers, rationales for correct and some incorrect responses, client needs categories, nursing process, and specialty areas follow each examination. A computer practice disk with 100 questions is supplied.

Comments

Strengths: Good test-taking information.
             Organized by content areas.

Weaknesses: Some questions too easy.

Question and Answer Books

Lippincott's Review for the NCLEX-PN, 4/e $28.95

Timby, B. & Scherer, J.

J. B. Lippincott, 484 pages, 8 1/2" × 11", 1994, ISBN 0-397-55024-3

Description: This book contains an introduction and four units. The introduction describes the organization of the NCLEX-PN examination, ways to prepare for it, and test-taking strategies to use. The first unit tests the mental health client needs; the next, maternity and newborn needs; the third unit, pediatric needs; and the final unit, medical–surgical disorders. Fourteen tests are included with these four sections, ranging from 91 to 140 questions, followed by two comprehensive examinations. The rationale section for each test includes the correct answer, rationales for correct and incorrect answers, nursing process and category of client needs being tested, and a test result grid. A computer practice disk with 100 questions is supplied.

Comments

Strengths: Rationales for correct responses are good.
Answers are at the end of each section.

Weaknesses: Rationales for incorrect responses need more depth.
Some questions too easy.

American Nursing Review Questions & Answers for NCLEX-PN $23.95

Healy, P.

Springhouse Corporation, 186 pages, 8 1/2" × 11", 1996, ISBN 0-87434-800-5

Description: This book contains five sections plus a post-test. The first section presents information about understanding the NCLEX-PN examination. It discusses the test plan, ways to prepare, and test-taking strategies to employ. Each question in the examination in the psychiatric, pediatric, obstetric, and medical–surgical nursing specialty areas is accompanied by the correct answer, rationales for correct and incorrect answers, category of client needs, nursing process, and level of difficulty. Two post-tests are offered at the end, which are followed by the correct answers, rationales for correct and incorrect answers, categories of client needs, nursing processes, and levels of difficulty. A computer practice disk is not supplied.

Comments

Strengths: Good level of questions.
Rationales are directly next to each question.

Weaknesses: Rationales need more information.
Rationales are directly next to each question.

The Chicago Review Press NCLEX-PN Practice and Review Test $15.95

B-

Waide, L. & Roland, B.

Chicago Review Press, 166 pages, 8 1/2" × 11", 1995, ISBN 1-55652-256-8

Description: This book contains an introduction, three practice tests, and the answers to the tests. The introduction includes a discussion of how the NCLEX-PN examination is designed, the advantages of a computerized examination, and how the examination is corrected and analyzed. It also describes the process of licensure for the practical/vocational nurse. The three practice tests contain 80 questions and are presented in a single-item format. The practice tests are presented in a comprehensive design. The answer sections include the correct answer and rationales for the correct response, rationales for some incorrect responses, nursing process category, and category of client needs. A computer practice disk with 100 questions is supplied.

Comments

Strengths: Questions are presented in CAT format.
            Easy to read.

Weaknesses: Lacks rationales for incorrect responses.
              Rationales need more depth.

Mosby's Q & A for NCLEX-PN $19.95

C+

Yannes-Eyles, M.

Mosby, 248 pages, 8 1/2" × 11", 1994, ISBN 0-8016-6952-9

Description: This book contains seven sections. The first section contains information about the NCLEX-PN examination, ways to prepare for it, and strategies for answering questions. The medical–surgical testing section is presented in a systems approach format which also includes fundamentals, geriatrics, and pharmacology questions. Questions about care of children are provided in the section on maternal–child nursing, which is followed by a psychiatric–mental health nursing section. One section is devoted to providing two comprehensive examinations followed by sections that present the correct answers, rationales for correct and incorrect answers, level of difficulty of questions, nursing process, and category of client needs. A computer practice disk is not supplied.

Comments

Strengths: Good rationales for questions.
            Provides rationales for correct and incorrect responses.

Weaknesses: Difficult to locate correct answers and rationales.
              Print is small.

Question and Answer Books

PART VI

▶ NCLEX-PN Practice Examination

- Questions
- Rationales for Questions
- References

This examination has been created to offer you some practice in answering questions that are similar in design to the actual examination. The test has been structured in the same manner as the NCLEX-PN examination. It contains 205 questions, which is the maximum number you will receive on your computerized examination. The questions have been developed using the same categories the National Council of State Boards of Nursing use and include:

Phases of the Nursing Process

- Data collection
- Planning
- Implementation
- Evaluation

Client Needs

- Safe, effective care environment
- Physiologic integrity
- Psychosocial integrity
- Health promotion and maintenance

The practice examination is followed by the correct answers and rationales for the correct and incorrect responses. In addition, the phase of nursing process and categories of client needs are highlighted. Finally, each answer is referenced with a specific source so you may go back to the book cited to obtain additional information and to see how the correct answer is supported by the literature (this is the method used by the NCLEX item writers to support their answers). This final portion is important, as it provides a direction for additional studying in areas in which you may not be particularly strong.

If you are taking this examination as a test of your ability, time yourself while you are testing and try to limit yourself to no more than one minute per question. Also, it is advisable **not** to take the examination one question at a time and then look up the answer. This type of practice will not allow you to get into a test-taking rhythm, because you are constantly stopping after each question to look at the answer. I recommend that if you are not going to take the entire examination all at once, then use it in blocks of 20 to 25 questions minimally. By spending at least 20 to 30 minutes testing, you can begin to establish a rhythm of multiple choice testing and can better balance your time in practice. You may notice that some questions in this examination appear similar; this is by design. During the actual NCLEX-PN, you may get a number of questions that appear similar. It does not mean you answered the previous questions incorrectly.

Proceed now to the first question, and I wish you

Good Luck and Good Testing!

1. Mr. Peters had an exploratory laparotomy today. In order to minimize muscular tension over his incision site, a binder is applied. This binder is described as

    A. a stretch net binder
    B. a T binder
    C. a straight abdominal binder
    D. an obstetric binder

2. When assisting a client following a cerebrovascular accident (CVA) to ambulate, the nurse would

    A. encourage the person to walk on his or her own.
    B. stand next to the person on the unaffected side.
    C. encourage the client to lift both feet to the same height.
    D. stay on the affected side of the person.

3. Which of the following would constitute a lack of understanding of universal precautions?

    A. wearing gloves while wiping a client's bloody nose
    B. wearing gloves while changing linen for a client with a large pressure sore
    C. wearing gloves while passing meal trays to clients with tuberculosis
    D. wearing gloves when assisting a client to the bathroom to void

4. Which of the following interventions would be contraindicated when administering oxygen to a client with chronic obstructive pulmonary disease (COPD)?

    A. applying moisturizers to the nares QID
    B. administering oxygen at 5 liters per minute
    C. displaying oxygen-in-use signs outside the room
    D. instructing the client that oxygen is considered an accelerant for fires

5. Which of the following would a person with hypothyroidism complain of?

    A. increased perspiration
    B. weight loss
    C. urinary incontinence
    D. constipation

6. A schizophrenic patient who has been taking an antipsychotic medication is observed with "lip smacking" behavior and some tremors. This is recognized as

    A. development of tardive dyskinesia.
    B. a hallucination response to voices giving him directions.
    C. a bizarre posturing affect.
    D. pseudo-convulsing from a tonic–clonic motor response.

7. Mr. Smith is being prepared for an endoscopic examination of the upper gastrointestinal tract. The nursing interventions will include

    A. holding any fluids until after the procedure.
    B. allowing sips of fluids until just prior to the procedure.
    C. having the client refrain from smoking until after the test.
    D. administering an antacid as part of the preprocedural prep.

8. Which of the following positions would be appropriate for insertion of a rectal suppository?

    A. dorsal lithotomy
    B. left lateral side-lying
    C. dorsal recumbent
    D. supine

9. Which of the following laboratory tests is used to measure the effectiveness of nutritional replacement?

    A. a serum potassium
    B. a serum sodium
    C. a folate level
    D. an albumin level

10. The reason females are more prone to urinary tract infections (UTIs) than males is attributed to the length of their

    A. ureters.
    B. urethra.
    C. pelvic bones.
    D. renal arteries.

11. While caring for a newborn infant, the nurse observes a circular swelling around the top of the baby's head. This is reported to the charge nurse and is described as

    A. caput succedaneum.
    B. cephalohematoma.
    C. erythema toxicum.
    D. bulging fontanel.

12. Which of the following assessments would be of **highest** priority in working with a client who has a plaster cast on his or her right leg?

    A. a warm feeling felt throughout the foot
    B. a tingling and numbness in the toes
    C. an intense itchiness under the cast
    D. a musty smell emanating from the cast

13. When managing a client in an emergency situation, which of the following has the **greatest** priority?

    A. airway maintenance
    B. cardiac status
    C. blood pressure assessment
    D. fluid replacement

14. When obtaining a urine sample from a catheter, the nurse can clamp the catheter for

    A. 5 minutes.
    B. 10 minutes.
    C. 30 minutes.
    D. 60 minutes.

15. While eating in the cafeteria, the nurse overhears several nursing assistants discussing the care of a specific client. Which of the following nursing actions would be **most** appropriate?

    A. Tell the nursing supervisor about this when the nurse returns to the unit.
    B. Go to the nursing assistants and tell them to stop talking about clients at the table.
    C. Confront the nursing assistants upon return to the unit after meal time.
    D. Report this breach of confidentiality to the client's family.

16. When would the nurse administer Carafate to a client with a peptic ulcer?

    A. 1/2 to 1 hour prior to meals
    B. while the client is eating
    C. 1/2 to 1 hour after meals
    D. at the time of sleep only

17. To evaluate whether an unconscious client is aspirating tube feedings, the nurse will

    A. dilute the feedings with normal saline.
    B. add food coloring to the feeding solution.
    C. monitor urinary output.
    D. check blood pressure before and after feeding.

18. Which of the following interventions may cause injury in a client with rheumatoid arthritis experiencing a flare-up (exacerbation) of the disease?

    A. encouraging active range of motion of the extremities
    B. positioning the client using splints and braces as designed
    C. performing passive range of motion exercises several times per day.
    D. medicating the client prior to any type of painful activities

19. When given to a client who has a history of angina and is complaining of a substernal chest pain rating 4 on a scale of 1 to 10, which of the following medications could cause a headache?

    A. propranolol hydrochloride (Inderal)
    B. acetaminophen (Tylenol)
    C. nitroglycerin
    D. morphine sulfate

20. The first step in obtaining proper measurement of a client's weight is to

    A. establish the height of the client.
    B. assure that privacy is maintained.
    C. balance the scale.
    D. have the client remove his or her clothes.

21. When caring for a child taking phenytoin sodium (Dilantin), the nurse would expect the urinary output to

    A. be pink-tinged in color.
    B. test glucose positive.
    C. increase immediately.
    D. become more frequent.

22. Mr. Jones, hospitalized on the inpatient psychiatric unit, has agreed to be interviewed by the nurse. As he is about to sit down to begin the interview, he asks, "What's going to happen now?" Which of the following represents the **best** response?

    A. "You decide what you'd like to talk about."
    B. "You seem worried about what's going to happen; tell me why you are worried and any specific concerns you have about our interview."
    C. "I saw in your chart that you're suicidal. Tell me about that."
    D. "I'm going to sit with you for about 30 minutes and talk to you about what brought you to the hospital and what you would like to happen while you are here."

23. When working with a client receiving a sitz bath, which of the following interventions would **not** be included in the plan?

    A. maintaining a water temperature of 98 to 102°F to promote healing.
    B. limiting the duration of the sitz bath to no more than 10 minutes.
    C. observing the client for signs of weakness or dizziness.
    D. staying with the client or placing a call bell within easy reach.

24. Mary Louise is admitted to the hospital after a sudden onset of blindness. A physical examination is negative. She tells the nurse that last night she witnessed the stabbing death of her best friend. This type of response is known as

A. reaction formation.
B. transference.
C. suppression.
D. conversion reaction.

25. Mr. Shear was admitted for management of congestive heart failure and suddenly developed acute pulmonary edema. Which of the following interventions would be **most** appropriate for this client?

A. Stay with the client and sit him up to assist in breathing.
B. Stay with the client and cover him with towels for diaphoresis.
C. Stay with the client and have him lie down in the shock position.
D. Stay with the client and count his pulse every 15 minutes.

26. A 77-year-old woman suffered a left-sided CVA, resulting in a right hemiparesis. To preserve her skin integrity, the nurse would plan to

A. position her at least every four hours.
B. massage pressure areas at least once per day.
C. encourage foods that are high in protein.
D. shower her daily in a special chair.

27. Which of the following would indicate that the client understands the management plan for treating a duodenal ulcer?

A. "I know I can never have alcohol again."
B. "I think most ulcers are caused by stress."
C. "I must drink fluids between meals only."
D. "I should eat small meals more frequently."

28. The **most** important consideration when working with older adult clients is to evaluate their

A. occupational history.
B. developmental stage.
C. social relationships.
D. economic independence.

29. Which of the following interventions would be **most** appropriate when working to improve the nutritional status of a client with a manic disorder during the manic phase?

A. dining with the client to provide an appropriate role model
B. serving meals when the client's energy is at its lowest point
C. providing foods such as sandwiches that can be eaten while moving
D. encouraging the client to assist in the preparation of his or her meals

30. Which of the following have the **greatest** exposure potential to hepatitis B?

A. people who travel to countries with poor sanitation
B. people who work with blood and blood products
C. people who care for children in day care centers
D. people who work in jails or prisons

31. *Wheezes, gurgles, and rattling lung sounds accompanied by dyspnea and a need to sit up are signs of*

    A. right-sided congestive heart failure.
    B. left-sided congestive heart failure.
    C. double pneumonia.
    D. emphysema.

32. *While observing a client experiencing a generalized tonic–clonic seizure, the nurse notes the muscles becoming very tight and tense. This is described as the*

    A. ictal phase of the seizure.
    B. clonic phase of the seizure.
    C. tonic phase of the seizure.
    D. onset phase of the seizure.

33. *Which of the following actions would be **most** appropriate for management of anxiety in a client undergoing a diagnostic test?*

    A. The nurse emphasizes that the test will not provide any form of treatment.
    B. The nurse notes that the procedure will be done in the early morning.
    C. The nurse explains what the client can expect to happen during the test.
    D. The nurse assures the client that the procedure will determine the extent of health problems.

34. *Jason Anderson is a 3-day post-radical prostatectomy surgical client who has just requested pain medication. His last pain medication administered was meperidine (Demerol) 75 mg with hydroxyzine (Vistaril) 25 mg intramuscularly 8 hours ago. At this point, the nurse would*

    A. administer another dose of meperidine and hydroxyzine per order.
    B. further assess the level of pain before medicating.
    C. obtain an order for an oral analgesic such as oxycodone (Percocet).
    D. have him focus on relaxation techniques.

35. *Kim is 15 years old and has had bulimia nervosa for 2 years. She asks the nurse if the damage she has done to her body is permanent. What would be the **most** therapeutic reply?*

    A. "It could be, I'm not sure."
    B. "What do you think?"
    C. "What caused you to ask that question?"
    D. "That's a very good question; perhaps we can ask the physician."

36. *Which of the following would be of **greatest** benefit for airway clearance when working with a post-thoracotomy client?*

    A. instructing the client to move about as soon as possible
    B. teaching the client how to splint the chest when taking deep breaths
    C. having the family members encourage the client to sit up
    D. ensuring that suction is at the bedside of the client

37. *Time periods are used to distinguish the difference between acute and chronic pain. Chronic pain is defined as a pain occurring longer than*

    A. 1 week.
    B. 1 month.
    C. 5 months.
    D. 12 months.

38. Which of the following positions is **most** likely to cause shortness of breath in a COPD client?

A. high-Fowler's position
B. Trendelenburg's position
C. sitting in a forward position
D. semi-Fowler's position

39. Mrs. Finnegan has been diagnosed with breast cancer. While doing morning care, the nurse asks her how she is feeling about her diagnosis. She tells the nurse, "I just have a cyst; you must be confusing me with another person." The defense mechanism she is using is

A. projection.
B. repression.
C. denial.
D. fantasy.

40. Which of the following would **most likely** indicate that a postoperative client is not physically tolerating walking down the hallway? The client

A. complains about feeling weak and tired.
B. expresses a feeling of nausea.
C. has a radial pulse of 140 beats per minute.
D. possesses a systolic pressure of 110 mm Hg.

41. When a client is thoroughly convinced that his wife is trying to kill him, in spite of evidence to the contrary, he is considered to be

A. delusional.
B. hallucinating.
C. having an illusion.
D. creating symbolism.

42. During the care of a postoperative gastrectomy client, the surgical wound separates, exposing the abdominal viscera. The nurse should

A. inform the surgeon immediately.
B. call for help while applying a dry, sterile dressing over the wound.
C. support the viscera to keep it from protruding.
D. cover the wound with a saline-soaked, sterile dressing.

43. Which of the following interventions would have the **highest** priority in a pediatric client experiencing a rapid pulse, tachypnea, and cool, clammy skin? The nurse would immediately

A. notify the charge nurse about the findings.
B. inform the client's family about the condition.
C. start oxygen at 5 liters per minute.
D. call a code and notify the primary physician.

44. Which of the following is considered an **early** sign of shock?

A. a pulse rate of 120
B. a blood pressure of 110/70
C. a respiratory rate of 24
D. a fever of 101°F

45. Which of the following methods would be **most** appropriate to identify a nursing home client who has lost his or her identification band?

A. Ask the client's roommate.
B. Check with a fellow nurse.
C. Ask the client his or her name.
D. Check the client's record.

46. When setting up a client for dinner, it is **most** important for the nurse to ensure that

A. the client has the foods he or she requested.
B. the tray has the client's name on it.
C. the proper diet has been ordered for the client.
D. the client is seated in an appropriate height chair.

47. During the suctioning of a client, the wall suction seems to become ineffective. The nurse should

A. recheck all connections.
B. notify the supervisor.
C. contact the plant manager.
D. shut the system down.

48. While turning and moving a client up in bed, the nurse would instruct nursing assistants to avoid

A. creating contractures.
B. soiling the linen.
C. changing the pull sheet.
D. creating shearing force.

49. Which of the following is considered a nursing intervention?

A. applying pressure over an area of bleeding
B. observing for signs of edema
C. checking for evidence of discharge in wounds
D. determining the needs of the family system

50. When developing a plan of personal hygiene, which of the following clients would have a complete bath every other day?

A. a 6-year-old child
B. a 22-year-old adult
C. a 45-year-old adult
D. a 74-year-old adult

51. Which of the following principles would be **most** significant in monitoring weight changes?

A. weighing the client after administration of diuretics
B. weighing the client wearing his or her regular clothes
C. weighing the client at the same time every day
D. weighing the client immediately prior to meals

52. A client diagnosed with congestive heart failure (CHF) is noted to have gained 4 1/2 pounds in the past 24 hours. The nurse would note this weight gain consistent with

A. 1 liter of fluid retention.
B. 2 liters of fluid retention.
C. 3 liters of fluid retention.
D. 4 liters of fluid retention.

53. When planning care for a client who has just had electroconvulsive therapy (ECT), which of the following would **most likely** be expected? The client

A. will not be depressed but will have a high suicide risk.
B. will want to be left alone to cry or sleep.
C. will be incontinent of urine and stool.
D. will be confused and may experience memory loss.

54. Which of the following complaints would indicate that the temperature of a sitz bath should be rechecked?

A. "I am having some perineal discomfort."
B. "I am feeling a little lightheaded."
C. "I think this may be causing constipation."
D. "I feel tingling in my perineal area."

55. To assist the left CVA client out of bed, the nurse would place the wheelchair

A. facing the client's right side.
B. perpendicular to the client's bed.
C. facing the client's left side.
D. at a 45-degree angle to the bed.

56. The proper method of administering an enema includes positioning the client

A. on his or her left side.
B. in the semi-recumbent position.
C. on his or her right side.
D. in the semi-Fowler's position.

57. When applying antithrombotic stockings to a client, which of the following measurements would **not** be required?

A. calf size
B. client weight
C. foot size
D. ankle size

58. Jody, a hospitalized 6-month-old child, began crying after a blood test was performed. Which of the following nursing interventions would be **most** appropriate?

A. recording this episode of crying
B. medicating her immediately
C. encouraging her mother to hold her
D. giving her a pacifier to suck on

59. The proper temperature for administration of a tepid sponge is

A. 70°F.
B. 80°F.
C. 90°F.
D. 100°F.

60. When performing perineal care on an uncircumcised male's penis, the nurse should return the foreskin to its natural position to prevent

A. an abnormal erection response.
B. localized swelling and edema.
C. potential urinary tract infection.
D. embarrassment of the client.

61. To assist in orienting a confused nursing home client, the plan will include

   A. constantly reminding the client that he is no longer at home.
   B. placing the client in group therapy with other confused clients.
   C. marking the door to the client's room with his name.
   D. placing the client near the nursing station during shift report.

62. Which of the following fruits would the nurse question giving the child with renal disease?

   A. apples
   B. bananas
   C. grapes
   D. pears

63. When establishing a sterile field for a sterile procedure, the nurse would open the sterile towel/drape

   A. toward his or her body first.
   B. away from his or her body first.
   C. to the left side of his or her body first.
   D. to the right side of his or her body first.

64. The proper placement of an abdominal binder on the postpartum cesarean section client will have the upper edge

   A. above the xiphoid process.
   B. at the level of the tenth rib.
   C. at the symphysis pubis.
   D. below the costal margins.

65. In a pediatric client undergoing a lumbar puncture, the nursing role is to

   A. keep the child in bed for 8 hours prior to the procedure.
   B. hold the child in the knee–chest position during the procedure.
   C. assure the child's parents that the procedure is harmless.
   D. record the child's vital signs throughout the procedure.

66. To obtain a 24-hour urine sample, the nurse would ensure that the client

   A. has taken at least 3 liters of fluids.
   B. keeps the indwelling catheter in place.
   C. understands the need to void hourly.
   D. voided just prior to the end of the collection.

67. Which of the following vital sign changes would require immediate intervention?

   A. a blood pressure of 140/88
   B. a pulse rate of 100
   C. a temperature of 98.8°F
   D. a respiratory rate of 36

68. Which of the following assessments would have the **highest** priority in cast care?

   A. assessing mental status and ability to communicate pain
   B. educating the client about how to maintain the cast properly
   C. considering the client's threshold for pain prior to casting
   D. evaluating for color, sensation, and motion of the casted extremity

69. The **most** important instruction to give a client regarding the collection of a urine specimen for measurement of glucose and ketones would be to

A. maintain a sterile approach throughout the collection.
B. place the container at the bedside after voiding.
C. wipe the perineal area with a disinfectant prior to the test.
D. void once prior to the collection of the actual specimen.

70. Which of the following findings in the urinalysis report would the nurse question as being abnormal?

A. straw-colored urine
B. glucose negative
C. blood negative
D. specific gravity of 1.001

71. Which statement indicates the need for additional teaching of a client who needs to apply an ice pack for a sprained ankle?

A. "I should keep the leg elevated whenever possible."
B. "The pack should be padded with a towel or cloth."
C. "The cold pack should be applied once per day."
D. "I should expect some swelling even after the application."

72. Which of the following types of hallucinations is **most** commonly associated with schizophrenia?

A. gustatory
B. auditory
C. tactile
D. olfactory

73. Which of the following interventions is **most** appropriate to assist a pediatric client taking liquid ferrous sulfate (iron)?

A. mixing the medication with milk and chocolate flavor
B. adding a flavoring the child likes to the solution
C. telling the child that the medication is like a liquid candy
D. diluting the medication and administering it via a straw

74. A client who has been diagnosed with kyphosis will possess

A. a flattening of the lumbar curve.
B. an increased convex curve in the thoracic vertebrae.
C. a lateral deviation of the spine.
D. a deviation in the sternocleidomastoid muscles.

75. When assisting a client from a bed to a chair for the first time postoperatively, the nurse would make sure to place the chair

A. at the head of the bed.
B. facing the bed.
C. at the foot of the bed.
D. against the wall.

76. Pat is a 23-year-old client who always makes the nurse feel very uncomfortable when interacting with her, as she stands extremely close to the nurse. This discomfort is most likely caused by

A. Pat's feeling of sexual attraction for the nurse.
B. the nurse's feeling physically intimidated by Pat.
C. her invasion into the nurse's personal space.
D. the nurse's unconscious wish to avoid her.

77. Which of the following precautions would be required when providing direct care to a client who has been recently diagnosed with pulmonary tuberculosis?

   A. gown and mask
   B. gloves and mask
   C. gown and gloves
   D. gown only

78. Which of the following would the nurse do **first** when a toxic exposure has occurred on the client unit?

   A. Inform the nurse in charge of the unit.
   B. Remove the clients from any immediate harm.
   C. Notify the fire department.
   D. Contact the environmental director.

79. Which of the following statements would be described as a component of a client's past health history?

   A. "I had an appendectomy in 1994."
   B. "My father died of lung cancer."
   C. "I worked in a dry cleaner for 25 years."
   D. "I graduated from high school when I was 18."

80. Which of the following client statements would indicate the need for additional teaching regarding prevention of constipation? "I will make sure to

   A. drink 2500 to 3000 mL of liquid each day."
   B. maintain a low-residue diet."
   C. eat three regular meals that include the four basic food groups."
   D. exercise several times per week for at least 20 minutes."

81. A client informs the nurse that she wishes to be left alone, saying, "I'm no good to anybody. Why don't you attend to someone who matters?" Which of the following responses would be the **most** therapeutic?

   A. "You are my client and I will stay with you."
   B. "I'm going to stay with you for the next 15 minutes."
   C. "Don't put yourself down like that, you are a good person."
   D. "Why do you think you are no good to anyone?"

82. Which of the following ostomies would **most likely** have an order to be irrigated?

   A. an ileostomy
   B. an ascending colostomy
   C. a sigmoid colostomy
   D. a transverse colostomy

83. Which of the following would indicate a lack of knowledge in a client performing a capillary blood sugar test?

   A. applying alcohol over the finger and waiting for it to dry
   B. using the lancet to puncture the fingertip/pad
   C. squeezing the finger for 5 minutes to obtain an ample amount of blood
   D. checking the machine prior to the test to ensure baseline information

84. The appropriate length of time to assess for respiratory arrest prior to starting CPR is between

A. 2 and 4 seconds.
B. 5 and 10 seconds.
C. 15 and 20 seconds.
D. 25 and 30 seconds.

85. Which of the following would the nurse do **first** after discovering a medication error?

A. Inform the patient.
B. Notify the charge nurse.
C. Call the doctor.
D. Recheck the order.

86. When evaluating a client for orientation, the nurse will **first** ask

A. where he is.
B. the date and year.
C. the time of day.
D. the person's name.

87. The reason children must be monitored to ensure completion of antibiotics for streptococcal throat infections is to prevent

A. pneumonia complications.
B. kidney disease complications.
C. liver failure complications.
D. brain abscess complications.

88. Working with a client experiencing mania requires the nurse to plan for

A. inclusion in reality orientation therapy programs.
B. impulsive actions and related safety issues.
C. periods of depression followed by suicidal ideation.
D. an increase in appetite and promiscuous sex acts.

89. Which of the following oxygen delivery systems would be **most** appropriate for the person with chronic airflow limitation (COPD)?

A. a nasal cannula
B. a simple face mask
C. a Venturi mask
D. a nonrebreathing mask

90. While observing a nursing assistant transfer a CVA client, the nurse notices that the wheelchair is placed on the client's affected side. The nurse would

A. remind the nursing assistant that the wheelchair should be placed on the unaffected side.
B. help the nursing assistant transfer the client from the bed to the wheelchair.
C. evaluate the effectiveness of the nursing assistant's actions for future performance evaluations.
D. ask the nursing assistant if additional help is needed in the transfer.

91. When inserting a rectal suppository, the nurse should

A. tell the client to relax during insertion.
B. stimulate the anal reflex prior to insertion.
C. have the client take a deep breath and hold it during insertion.
D. ask the client to bear down, as in moving the bowels, during insertion.

92. Which of the following complaints has the **greatest priority** for care in the person with benign prostatic hypertrophy?

A. urinary retention
B. burning on urination
C. dribbling of urine
D. decreased urine stream

93. Which of the following would **not** be included in the teaching plan to prevent hypoglycemic reactions in a diabetic client? Instructing the client to

A. call the doctor immediately if nausea, vomiting, or diarrhea occurs
B. not skip meals during the day and take supplements as ordered
C. make certain that the meal is served within 30 minutes after regular insulin is administered
D. observe for signs such as a hot, dry feeling experienced in late afternoon

94. A client complains of pain in the lower right quadrant of his abdomen. This represents information considered to be

A. objective data.
B. observable data.
C. summative data.
D. subjective data.

95. Which of the following interventions would help to prevent nipple soreness in the mother who is breast feeding her baby?

A. Tell the mother that nipple soreness can be controlled with acetaminophen.
B. Have the mother apply a lotion to the nipple at least four times per day.
C. Instruct the mother to remove the baby from the nipple every 1 minute.
D. Encourage the mother to place the majority of the areola into the baby's mouth.

96. When administering medications via a nasogastric tube, the nurse would first

A. aspirate to confirm placement in the stomach.
B. flush the tube with water.
C. push air in and auscultate over the stomach with a stethoscope.
D. administer only liquid medications.

97. Crohn's disease is characterized by

A. rectal bleeding and abdominal cramping.
B. diarrhea and intestinal fistulas.
C. right lower abdominal pain with rebound tenderness.
D. gastroesophageal reflux.

98. Which of the following medications would **not** be indicated for use as an antacid?

A. aluminum hydroxide
B. magnesium
C. bismuth
D. calcium carbonate

99. Mrs. Spang was admitted with a diagnosis of carcinoma of the esophagus. Which of the following would be an **early** complaint?

A. constipation
B. hematemesis
C. dysphasia
D. hoarseness

100. Which of the following would **not** require an ostomy appliance or bag?

  A. an ileal conduit
  B. a urostomy
  C. a transverse colostomy
  D. a Kock's pouch

101. The proper depth of chest compressions in adult CPR is

  A. 1/2 to 1 inch.
  B. 1 to $1^1/_2$ inches.
  C. $1^1/_2$ to 2 inches.
  D. 2 to $2^1/_2$ inches.

102. The signs and symptoms seen in the first trimester of pregnancy include Chadwick's sign. This sign is known as a

  A. presumptive sign of pregnancy.
  B. probable sign of pregnancy.
  C. positive sign of pregnancy.
  D. negative sign of pregnancy.

103. While observing a treatment nurse set up a sterile field, the licensed practical nurse notes that the person's shirt sleeve has lightly brushed the top of the sterile towel. The nurse would

  A. inform the treatment nurse that she has contaminated the field.
  B. suggest that the treatment nurse avoid a specific portion of the sterile field.
  C. tell the treatment nurse to wait, and leave the room to obtain a new sterile field.
  D. discuss the breach of sterility with the treatment nurse after the procedure.

104. While providing care for a stage 3 pressure sore, the nurse should apply the wet portion of the wet-to-dry dressing

  A. over the entire wound and the surrounding skin to create a barrier.
  B. on the necrotic area only to ensure adherence.
  C. over the inside portion of the wound to prevent maceration.
  D. on the healthy tissue within the ulcer to improve circulation.

105. Mrs. Sandra Wilson, a 91-year-old nursing home resident, has been confused since 7 o'clock in the evening. She is trying to get out of bed and go home. The nurse would

  A. administer chloral hydrate (Noctec) as ordered.
  B. encourage Mrs. Wilson to try some reading.
  C. call her husband at home and have him come in.
  D. notify the charge nurse of this mental status change.

106. Which of the following observations is consistent with absence (or petite mal) seizure activity?

  A. a daydreaming-like appearance not responsive to commands
  B. a sudden loss of consciousness and fall to the floor
  C. a spasm of the extremities described as a tonic–clonic reaction
  D. a sudden jerking motion followed by loss of consciousness

107. When teaching a client about a computed tomography (CT) scan of the abdomen, which of the following would indicate a need for further teaching? The client reports that

  A. the procedure will last from 15 to 45 minutes.
  B. he will be placed within a closed area.
  C. he will not feel any pain during the procedure.
  D. he will be asked to move around during the procedure.

108. Which of the following positions would ensure the **best** airway for a client having difficulty breathing?

A. the side-lying position
B. the prone position
C. the Fowler's position
D. the supine position

109. Upon entering a client's room, the nurse observes the nursing assistant bathing a comatose client. The assistant leaves the client uncovered while obtaining more warm water. Which of the following actions would the nurse take?

A. Close the door to provide privacy and return later.
B. Advise the nursing assistant to cover the client after the bath.
C. Report the nursing assistant to the charge nurse for keeping the client uncovered during the bed bath.
D. Instruct the nursing assistant to cover the client immediately, exposing only one portion of the body at a time.

110. The use of incentive spirometry is important in postoperative clients and those on bedrest to prevent

A. pulmonary edema.
B. atelectasis.
C. pneumothorax.
D. pulmonary embolism.

111. Which of the following problems would the nurse report immediately when observed in a client with diabetes mellitus?

A. a complaint of decreased appetite
B. a fruity odor to the client's breath
C. a decrease in urinary output
D. a craving for sweets

112. A newborn with a decreased immune system will **most likely** be affected by

A. urinary tract infections.
B. candidal infections of the mouth.
C. skin lesions of varying colors.
D. bleeding and severe anemia.

113. Which of the following signs would a client suffering from hypovolemic shock present with first?

A. confusion
B. bradycardia
C. hypotension
D. loss of consciousness

114. The family of Drew Rogers, a cardiac client, ask what foods are good sources of potassium for replacement during diuretic therapy. Which of the following suggestions would provide the **least** amount of potassium?

A. bananas
B. orange juice
C. bran cereals
D. skim milk

115. The nurse discovers a gap of four empty lines in the progress notes between the progress note he has entered and the prior entry. The nurse would

A. know that this is not a problem as long as he records the correct time, date, and shift on his entry.

B. use the space to add a new entry in later in the day.

C. draw a straight line from the previous entry to the new entry to fill in the space.

D. remove the page and rewrite the entries according to times, leaving no space between entries.

116. Mrs. Franchi has been admitted with pericarditis. The **best** position to facilitate her breathing would be to place her

A. in the prone position.

C. onto her left side.

B. in a low-Fowler's position.

D. in an upright position.

117. Mr. Fiore, a nursing home resident, has been alert and oriented throughout the day. At 3 P.M. the nurse hears him say "I've lived in this house for 25 years." The next action taken by the nurse should be to

A. ask more questions to assess his mental status.

B. check his oxygen saturation level.

C. call the physician and notify him of this change.

D. refer to his chart to check lab values.

118. Mr. Smith initiates the universal choke sign at the dinner table. After confirming that he is choking, the nurse would

A. assess Mr. Smith's pulse and ability to speak.

B. lie him down and perform abdominal thrusts.

C. perform four to five back blows immediately on Mr. Smith.

D. approach him from behind and perform abdominal thrusts.

119. Client teaching for the use of medication to treat acute pain should include instructing the client to self-administer the medication

A. whenever the pain becomes moderate to severe.

B. after any procedure or activity that would induce the pain.

C. when the pain begins to become apparent to the client.

D. on a regular basis four to six times per day.

120. Which of the following would indicate a problem with the patency of a gastrostomy tube?

A. The nurse aspirates only 5 mL of stomach contents.

B. The nurse is unable to inject air into the tube.

C. Blood is coming from the tube opening.

D. The return aspirate is full of a green bile-like substance.

121. Which of the following would the nurse do **first** to facilitate proper drainage of a urinary catheter?

A. Maintain the height of all tubing lower than the level of the bladder and urethra.

B. Attach the bag to the side of the bed when the client is sitting up.

C. Affix the collection bag to an intravenous pole during ambulation.

D. Have the client hold the drainage bag at the waist level while ambulating.

122. *Prior to a magnetic resonance imaging (MRI) scan, the nurse must determine if the client*

   A. has a calcium allergy.
   B. has a pacemaker.
   C. has signed an operative consent form.
   D. knows the method of recovery from the test.

123. *During the initial phase of trauma, a rape victim will often be found to be*

   A. in total denial that the event occurred.
   B. attempting to compensate by using fantasy.
   C. wanting to repeat the story to relive the event.
   D. in a state of shock and guilt.

124. *When performing a subcutaneous injection on a 6-year-old child, the nurse would select a needle that is*

   A. 25 gauge, 1/2 inch long.
   B. 22 gauge, 3/4 inch long.
   C. 19 gauge, 1 inch long.
   D. 17 gauge, $1\frac{1}{2}$ inches long.

125. *Which of the following would help ensure a correct blood pressure reading?*

   A. using a very narrow bladder and cuff
   B. keeping the cuff wrapped very loosely
   C. deflating the cuff over 1 to 2 minutes
   D. using a calibrated manometer

126. *When teaching a client to use a walker, the nurse would instruct the client to move the walker*

   A. 6 inches ahead at a time.
   B. 12 inches ahead at a time.
   C. 18 inches ahead at a time.
   D. 24 inches ahead at a time.

127. *A developmental delay could be indicated in an 8-month-old infant who is unable to*

   A. stand while holding on to furniture.
   B. crawl a short distance.
   C. sit alone using hands for support.
   D. creep on hands and knees.

128. *Which of the following would be considered unsafe when using a Hoyer lift to transfer a client from bed to chair?*

   A. pumping the hydraulic handle, using slow, long, even strokes until the client is raised off the bed
   B. folding the client's arms over his or her chest during the transfer
   C. releasing the check valve in a quick fashion to lower the client into the chair
   D. ensuring that the straps are secured onto the lift prior to the lifting process

129. *A child with epispadias would have difficulty*

   A. speaking.
   B. sitting.
   C. walking.
   D. voiding.

130. After knee replacement surgery a client is placed on a continuous passive motion device (CPM). The purpose of this device is to

A. promote healing of the knee joint and increase circulation to the operative site.
B. decrease extension and flexion of the joint to prevent any additional bleeding.
C. prevent atrophy of the muscles on the nonoperative side.
D. keep the leg in an abducted position, creating isometric strengthening.

131. Mr. Adams' blood pressure is 150/86. He is concerned that he has hypertension and has a positive family history of it. During education, he will be informed that hypertension is defined as a sustained pressure over

A. 120/70.
B. 140/90.
C. 120/80.
D. 130/70.

132. When instructing a pregnant client to take iron replacement as ordered by the physician, the nurse would advise her to administer the medication

A. 1 hour prior to eating breakfast.
B. while she is eating a meal.
C. 1 hour after she has eaten.
D. immediately prior to going to bed.

133. Which of the following would indicate a need for **additional** teaching of a diabetic regarding measuring capillary blood glucose levels? The client

A. uses the large droplet of blood formed immediately after the puncture.
B. holds the reagent strip test pad close to the drop of blood and lightly transfers the droplet to the test pad.
C. does not smear the blood on the test pad.
D. presses the timer immediately on the glucose meter and places the reagent strip on a paper towel at the side of the timer.

134. Which of the following would the nurse use to collect data about the "aura" experienced by a seizure client?

A. "Do you have any indications that a seizure is coming on?"
B. "Do you have difficulty breathing during the seizure?"
C. "Are you able to awaken without problems after the seizure?"
D. "Can you describe how the seizure occurs from beginning to end?"

135. Which of the following positions would be **most** appropriate for a client suffering from a left-sided CVA?

A. positioning the client on the abdomen
B. positioning the client on the back
C. positioning the client on the unaffected side
D. positioning the client on the affected side

136. Which of the following IV sites would be **most** appropriate for a client requiring additional fluid replacement?

A. the arm that has just recently had the IV running in it
B. the extremity that has not received recent fluids
C. the arm into which blood is being transfused
D. the extremity that has a saline lock in place with a continuous medication drip

137. Mr. Chase has become upset regarding an incident with a staff member that occurred 2 weeks ago. When speaking to him, the nurse should focus the conversation on

A. changing the subject to focus on the present day's activities.
B. recognizing that the patient may be confused and will probably become violent.
C. seeking to identify the actual source of the client's concern.
D. confronting the client and asking him directly what is wrong.

138. Which of the following would be appropriate for helping a 6-year-old child cope with hospitalization?

A. providing the child with a pull toy
B. giving the child a blood pressure cuff
C. assisting with a 300-piece puzzle
D. getting a telephone in the room

139. When caring for a client with emphysema, the nurse could expect complaints of

A. shortness of breath with minimal exertion.
B. a nonproductive cough.
C. increased appetite and a gain in weight.
D. an inability to sleep during the day.

140. Which antacid would be the **most** likely to cause diarrhea?

A. calcium carbonate
B. magnesium
C. aluminum
D. simethicone

141. The physician ordered an enema for Mr. Spencer to relieve gastric distention. The type of enema ordered is known as

A. a physiologic normal saline enema.
B. a soap suds enema.
C. an oil retention enema.
D. a carminative enema.

142. The type of respiration characterized by alternating periods of apnea and deep, rapid breathing is described as

A. dyspneic.
B. Kussmaul.
C. Cheyne–Stokes.
D. orthopneic.

143. When instructing a postpartum client about Kegel exercises, the nurse would explain that the exercises will

A. help to minimize episodes of constipation.
B. reverse any form of rectal prolapse.
C. allow the bladder to fight off infections.
D. assist in pelvic muscle healing and strength.

144. Which of the following would be considered an **early** sign of laryngeal cancer?

A. shortness of breath
B. recurrent pneumonia
C. coughing up blood
D. nagging hoarseness

145. Which of the following statements, made by the client's son, could indicate the potential that he is abusing his elderly father?

   A. "I feel as if I am somehow being punished for something."
   B. "It is difficult to keep reminding him of where he is."
   C. "I have found him wandering outside on a number of occasions."
   D. "His confusion seems to come and go."

146. Mrs. Ahearn is discovered to have a pressure ulcer that shows destruction of tissue involving subcutaneous layers. The internal diameter is larger than the surface appearance. This observation is consistent with a

   A. stage 1 ulcer.
   B. stage 2 ulcer.
   C. stage 3 ulcer.
   D. stage 4 ulcer.

147. When a client suffers a left-sided CVA, he or she will often present with

   A. confusion and lethargy.
   B. aphasia and inability to follow directions.
   C. left-sided hemiplegia with neglect.
   D. loss of consciousness and blindness.

148. Which of the following gaits would the nurse expect to see in a client with Parkinson's disease?

   A. a broad-base gait
   B. a shuffling–propulsive gait
   C. a steppage gait
   D. a hemiplegic gait

149. Crohn's disease is characterized by frequent episodes of

   A. nausea and vomiting.
   B. painful diarrhea.
   C. prolonged constipation.
   D. gastric bleeding.

150. When instructing a client on how to record on his or her intake and output (I&O) sheet, the nurse would advise the client that which of the following is **not** considered part of the intake of fluids?

   A. ice cream
   B. sips of water
   C. custards
   D. applesauce

151. When a nursing assistant ambulates a client with hemiplegia, which of the following would indicate unsafe practice? The nursing assistant

   A. stands next to the client's affected side and supports the client by grasping the safety belt in the middle of the client's back or one arm around the client's waist and the other arm around the inferior aspect of the client's upper arm.
   B. stands next to the client's unaffected side and supports the client by placing one arm around the client's waist and the other arm around the inferior aspect of the client's upper arm.
   C. takes a few steps forward with the client to assess for strength and balance.
   D. stands on the client's affected side while the client moves with a cane.

152. In which of the following positions would it be **most** appropriate to place a child with a meningomyelocele prior to surgical correction?

    A. a modified side-lying position
    B. the supine position
    C. the high-Fowler's position
    D. the prone position

153. When talking with a suicidal client, it is important to establish

    A. the presence of family support.
    B. whether or not he has a plan.
    C. his reason for committing suicide.
    D. the reason he feels the need to end his life.

154. When discussing urinary tract infections in females, the nurse would highlight

    A. the need for drinking several glasses of milk per day.
    B. eating foods which increase the alkalinity of urine.
    C. wiping from front to back after urination.
    D. limiting sexual intercourse.

155. The first day after delivery, a mother focuses on the birthing experience and does little for herself or her newborn. This would be considered part of the

    A. bonding phase.
    B. taking-hold phase.
    C. taking-in phase.
    D. letting-go phase.

156. Mrs. Sauls had a total hip replacement yesterday. In order to facilitate recovery, the nurse should

    A. elevate her legs on pillows and keep them in an adducted position.
    B. place the affected leg in traction and limit motion.
    C. position pillows or supports to maintain the hip in an abducted position.
    D. remove any braces, supports, or pillows while turning.

157. Which of the following questions would the nurse ask of a person undergoing a CT scan?

    A. "Do you have a history of hay fever?"
    B. "Do you have an allergy to shellfish?"
    C. "Are you allergic to MSG?"
    D. "Are you sensitive to any antibiotics?"

158. Bob Woodin, age 32, is complaining about his physician. He states, "My doctor is such an incompetent jerk." The **best** response to Mr. Woodin is

    A. "Give me an example of your doctor's incompetence."
    B. "Sometimes when we are feeling incompetent, we project that onto others."
    C. "I can't talk to you when you're criticizing your doctor."
    D. "You complain so much, it must be hard on your doctor to treat you."

159. Which of the following positions is contraindicated in a client who has just had surgical correction of a cleft lip?

    A. sitting in an infant seat
    B. lying prone with the mattress flat
    C. a side-lying position with supports
    D. a semi-Fowler's position

160. When working with a rape victim, the nurse should

   A. establish a therapeutic relationship with the client.
   B. have the client accept some responsibility for the act.
   C. help the client remember the details of the rape crisis.
   D. encourage the client to confront and report the rapist.

161. Scott was admitted to the mental health unit 3 weeks ago with a diagnosis of depression. He is improving and participating in treatment programs and is ready for discharge when he

   A. calls his employer and informs him of his readiness to return to work.
   B. is able to fully identify his strengths and express his anxieties.
   C. discusses plans to go home and continue treatment as an outpatient.
   D. can create a list of things he wants to change about himself.

162. A postoperative client's urine output has averaged over 400 mL per shift for the past 48 hours. After caring for the client for the last 2 hours, his nurse notes only 30 cc of urine in the bag. The nurse's **first** action would be to

   A. call the physician after looking up lab values of kidney function.
   B. observe the client's output over the next 2 hours and report.
   C. check all connections to the Foley catheter for patency or kinking.
   D. deflate the catheter balloon, reposition the catheter, and reinflate.

163. When an older client talks to the nurse about sexual thoughts and feelings, it most likely indicates that the patient is acting

   A. impulsively.
   B. inappropriately.
   C. normally.
   D. pervertedly.

164. The rationale for using antipsychotic drugs with schizophrenia is to relieve

   A. paranoia and hallucinations.
   B. a lack of personal identity.
   C. tremors and wandering.
   D. depressive behaviors.

165. Which of the following solutions would the nurse select when bottle feeding the newborn for the first time?

   A. a premixed formula
   B. a dextrose and saline solution
   C. a diluted milk formula
   D. sterile water

166. The primary goal for planning range of motion exercises with a client is to

   A. improve circulation.
   B. prevent the skin from breaking down.
   C. promote joint motion and flexibility.
   D. assist with ambulation.

167. Which of the following would **not** be included as part of the plan to implement universal precautions?

   A. Cap, gown, and mask are to be worn when handling items or surfaces soiled with blood or body fluids.
   B. Spills of blood or body fluids can be cleaned up with a 1:10 solution of bleach and water.
   C. Gloves must be worn for performing venipuncture and other vascular access procedures.
   D. Gloves will be worn when coming into contact with body fluids, mucous membranes, or open skin areas.

168. A 20-year-old client on a psychiatric unit tells the nurse, "You are the only one who listens to me. The other nurses on this unit hate me." This person is attempting to create

A. a fantasy world.
B. disorder and confusion.
C. splitting of the staff.
D. intellectualization.

169. A nurse is caring for a client with an obsessive–compulsive disorder. Which of the following behaviors would alert the nurse that the client is under an increasing level of stress?

A. a general withdrawal from reality
B. a greater use of ritualistic behavior
C. an inability to communicate without using neologisms
D. an aggressive and physically violent response

170. A 4-year-old child has been casted for a fractured radius. When evaluating circulation in the casted extremity, the finding requiring **immediate** notification of the physician is

A. a radial pulse of 100.
B. complaints of pain in the affected arm.
C. cold, pale fingers.
D. increasing irritability of the child.

171. Which of the following signs or symptoms would indicate a worsening in a client with a fluid volume deficit?

A. Edematous areas are noted throughout.
B. Pulmonary edema occurs.
C. The client becomes confused.
D. The client becomes hyperactive.

172. A 45-year-old woman is demanding of everyone and shows no concern for anyone but herself. Erickson would note that her stage of development is

A. intimacy versus isolation.
B. autonomy versus shame and doubt.
C. generativity versus stagnation.
D. identity versus role confusion.

173. While providing a partial bed bath to a client, the nurse should make sure to

A. wash one part of the body at a time.
B. wash the face, hands, and perineal area only.
C. assist the client in washing the face, hands, axillary areas, back, and perineal area.
D. direct the client to wash as much as he or she feels able, providing assistance to all other parts of the body.

174. The use of a nasogastric tube postoperatively is indicated to provide for gastric

A. gavage.
B. lavage.
C. decompression.
D. installations.

175. Which of the following symptoms or signs represents a toxemic state?

A. A pregnant woman gains 1 pound over the course of a week.
B. A client complains of a severe headache and has an increase in blood pressure.
C. An expectant mother develops backaches, fatigue, and a drop in blood pressure.
D. A client complains of heartburn, indigestion, and vomiting.

176. Which of the following represents the correct method for administration of a rectal suppository?

    A. Place the client prone and insert the suppository beyond the sphincter.

    B. Place the client on his or her left side, lubricate the suppository with a water-based lubricant, and insert it beyond sphincter.

    C. Place the client on his or her right side, lubricate the suppository with petroleum jelly, and insert it beyond the sphincter.

    D. Place the client in a semi-Fowler's position and insert the suppository beyond the sphincter.

177. Mrs. Gilbert is an insulin-dependent diabetic. She has a stage 3 ulcer on her left foot. Which of the following would be **unnecessary** prior to removing the dressing?

    A. having all the equipment ready to replace the dressing

    B. premedicating 1 to 1½ hours prior to applying the dressing

    C. setting up a sterile field

    D. obtaining vital signs

178. A sterile dressing, by definition, must be

    A. free of pathogens.

    B. free of pathogenic and nonpathogenic organisms.

    C. free of pathogenic and nonpathogenic organisms and their spores.

    D. free of all living and nonliving organisms.

179. When a client diagnosed with herpes genitalis becomes pregnant, she will need information about

    A. having sexual contact with multiple partners.

    B. the possibility of having a cesarean section.

    C. maintaining abstinence during the pregnancy.

    D. the increased incidence of gonorrhea.

180. For clients with severe thrombocytopenia, the bleeding precautions would include allowing them to

    A. shave with a regular razor.

    B. brush their teeth with a cotton-tipped swab.

    C. have their temperature taken rectally.

    D. eat a high-fiber diet with raw fruits.

181. Which of the following tests would be indicated to evaluate for AIDS?

    A. a serum albumin

    B. a white blood cell count

    C. a serum transferase and alkaline phosphatase

    D. an enzyme-linked immunosorbent assay

182. Which of the following information is important in determining a risk factor for a person who may develop herpes zoster?

    A. a history of recurrent viral infections

    B. a history of chickenpox infection

    C. a history of rheumatic fever

    D. a history of candidal infections

183. When determining the needs of clients, the nurse recognizes that Maslow's first level of needs to be met are the

    A. physiologic needs.
    B. safety and security needs.
    C. love and belonging needs.
    D. self-actualization needs.

184. When a client and nurse sign an informed consent permission form, the nurse's signature ensures that

    A. the client is of sound mind.
    B. the client is doing this voluntarily and knowledgeably.
    C. the nurse has informed the client of all consequences.
    D. the nurse actually witnessed the signing.

185. When caring for an AIDS client, the nurse notes a bluish-whitish plaque-like ulcer in the client's mouth. The nurse would inform the physician that the client may have developed

    A. Kaposi's sarcoma
    B. a candidal infection
    C. a pneumocystis infection
    D. a mycobacterial infection

186. Which of the following diagnostic tests would be of **greatest** significance when planning the care of a client on heparin?

    A. a white blood cell count
    B. an x-ray of the chest
    C. a stool sample for occult blood
    D. a serum potassium

187. Which of the following is important to do with older clients every morning?

    A. Wash each lens of their glasses.
    B. Determine if they have slept well.
    C. Ascertain their medication history.
    D. Give them a complete bath.

188. When planning the nutritional management of a person prescribed a low-residue diet, the nurse would make sure the client understands that he or she can have

    A. strained vegetables and fruits.
    B. hard-boiled or fried eggs.
    C. no milk or milk products.
    D. whole-grain cereals.

189. Which of the following liquids would an older person who needs potassium replacement be advised to drink?

    A. apple juice
    B. prune juice
    C. diet cola
    D. tonic water

190. When administering an intradermal injection, the nurse would hold the syringe at a

    A. 90-degree angle from the skin.
    B. 45-degree angle from the skin.
    C. 25-degree angle from the skin.
    D. 15-degree angle from the skin.

191. When caring for a child with cystic fibrosis, the nurse would expect the stools to
    A. be of a hard and formed consistency.
    B. be foul smelling and frothy.
    C. contain a small amount of fresh blood.
    D. test positive for ova and parasites.

192. Mr. Martin, a preoperative client, begins crying and becomes incoherent on the morning of the procedure and is attempting to leave. Physical problems have been ruled out. He would be described as experiencing a
    A. moderate level of anxiety.
    B. severe level of anxiety.
    C. tunnel vision level of anxiety.
    D. panic level of anxiety.

193. Which of the following would the nurse assess for in an infant who is ordered to have the MMR (measles, mumps, and rubella) vaccine?
    A. the developmental stage of the infant
    B. whether the child has an allergy to eggs
    C. the blood type of the child
    D. a history of hay fever to grasses and pollen

194. When instructing the parents of a newborn about developmental milestones, the nurse would highlight that these are
    A. used as a point of reference and are not absolute norms.
    B. the best guide to determine whether the child will grow.
    C. vague descriptions of what should be accomplished.
    D. have not been validated by research and are not reliable.

195. When instructing a pregnant client about average weight gain, the nurse would reinforce that the ideal gain is
    A. 5 to 15 pounds.
    B. 15 to 20 pounds.
    C. 25 to 30 pounds.
    D. 30 to 40 pounds.

196. Which of the following statements would the nurse use when trying to get the demented client, who is angrily arguing about where he is to come to dinner?
    A. "You are not at home and it's now time for supper."
    B. "You shouldn't get angry at me; I am just trying to give you dinner."
    C. "You are in the nursing home, and it is time for dinner."
    D. "You may not want to eat now, but it is dinnertime."

197. Which of the following nursing goals has the **highest** priority in the early postoperative recovery period for a client who has undergone a mastectomy?
    A. anxiety
    B. body image
    C. self-care deficit
    D. airway clearance

198. When working with a client with a skin disorder requiring a wet dressing, it is important to remember to

A. change the dressing every hour.
B. keep the dressing from drying out.
C. cover the dressing with a biologic dressing.
D. use only sterile water as the solution.

199. When wrapping the extremity of a client who has had an above-the-knee amputation, the nurse would start the bandage

A. around the waist.
B. on the thigh of the amputated leg.
C. just above the level of the amputation, moving in a figure-eight fashion.
D. on the calf of the amputated leg, proceeding with a figure-eight wrap.

200. Which of the following would be the **best** statement to stimulate a conversation with a client about his of her social history?

A. "Are you married?"
B. "Do you have any children?"
C. "Tell me about your family."
D. "Your role in the family is important."

201. When working with a depressed client, the nurse should make sure that the initial contacts

A. establish a trusting environment.
B. create a method of communication.
C. address the root cause of the depression.
D. do not depress the client any further.

202. Which of the following recommendations would be appropriate for a client who has undergone a cataract extraction with a lens replacement?

A. The client should lie flat in bed at night to prevent pressure buildup.
B. The client should wear an eye shield when sleeping.
C. The client should lie on the operative side at night.
D. The client will have an increased level of pain at night.

203. Which of the following medications would the nurse be likely to provide education for in the discharge plan of a client who has undergone a prostatectomy?

A. antiviral medications
B. antacid preparations
C. stool softeners
D. vitamin supplements

204. The use of long-term corticosteroids in conditions such as brain tumors will give rise to the problems associated with

A. Addison's disease.
B. Cushing's disease.
C. hyperthyroidism.
D. diabetes insipidus.

205. When caring for a client who is having a cast put on his or her leg, the nurse will make sure

A. that the client is able to move about without having to use any crutches or support.
B. that voiding is performed at least four times per day using a bedpan.
C. to handle the cast with the palms of the hands until it is completely dry.
D. that the family members know how to perform blood pressures and apical pulses.

1. **(C)** Correct. The straight abdominal binder centers support over abdominal structures. It provides continuous wound support and comfort. (A) Incorrect. A stretch net binder is used for support of dressings or surgical sites over the client's arms or legs. (B) and (D) Incorrect. The T and double T binders are applied to facilitate placement of perineal dressings and provide support to perineal muscles and organs. *Implementation/Physiologic Integrity (Ellis, Nowlis, and Bentz, 1996, p. 632)*

2. **(D)** Correct. To maximize client safety when ambulating, it is recommended that the nurse remain on the affected side of the client. This allows the client additional support and assists in maintaining an appropriate center of gravity. (A) Incorrect. This would not be a safe method of assisting the client. (B) Incorrect. Standing next to the person on their unaffected side will not allow the nurse to maximize assistance. (C) Incorrect. The person with a CVA will have a different type of gait and probably require additional ankle braces or supports. This client does not have a shuffling gait, so the focus would be directed more to balance and posture. *Implementation/Safe Environment (Ellis, Nowlis, and Bentz, 1996, p. 493)*

3. **(C)** Correct. The wearing of gloves while passing trays for tuberculosis clients is not necessary and is not part of the universal precaution procedure. (A), (B), and (D) Incorrect. These are all accepted standards in the universal precaution guidelines and should be employed whenever the nurse is exposed to body fluids and blood. *Implementation/Physiologic Integrity (Rosdahl, 1995, p. 336)*

4. **(B)** Correct. Administering oxygen at 5 liters per minute is too much oxygen for a person who has chronic lung disease. It will create respiratory arrest potential because these people respond to a hypoxic drive. (A), (C), and (D) Incorrect. All of these interventions would be recommended for the person receiving oxygen. *Implementation/Physiologic Integrity. (Christensen and Kockrow, 1995, p. 929)*

5. **(D)** Correct. As the individual's metabolic function begins to slow down, he or she will notice a decrease in bowel movements leading to constipation. (A) and (B) Incorrect. These would be seen in hyperthyroidism. (C) Incorrect. This has no direct association to either type of thyroid disease. *Data Collection/Physiologic Integrity (Thompson, McFarland, Hirsch, and Tucker, 1997, p. 831)*

6. **(A)** Correct. These symptoms are associated with this irreversible problem and are directly related to taking the psychotropic medication for too long a period. (B), (C), and (D) Incorrect. None of these are considered correct responses and are not associated with the condition described. *Data Collection/Psychosocial Integrity (Bailey and Bailey, 1993, p. 145)*

7. **(A)** Correct. To minimize the danger of aspiration, the client should not take any food or fluid after midnight or within 8 hours of the test. (B) Incorrect. There is a significant danger of aspiration. (C) Incorrect. The client should not smoke after the test, as it will increase their potential for a sore throat. (D) Incorrect. This could contribute to aspiration and pneumonia. *Data Collection/Physiological Integrity (Rosdahl, 1995, p. 1179)*

8. **(B)** Correct. The left lateral side-lying position exposes the anus and helps the client to relax the external anal sphincter. The left side lessens the likelihood of the suppository or feces being inadvertently expelled. (A) Incorrect. Dorsal lithotomy positioning is used for examination of the female genitalia. (C) and (D) Incorrect. Dorsal recumbent and supine are both positions with the client lying on his or her back. *Implementation/Physiologic Integrity (Perry and Potter, 1994, p. 536)*

9. **(D)** Correct. Albumin and protein measure the nutritional status of people. Low levels of either are consistent with malnutrition. (A) Incorrect. A serum potassium may be used to determine the effect of a diuretic on a client. (B) Incorrect. A serum sodium may be used to measure the fluid or hydration level of a client. (C) Incorrect. A folate level is used to evaluate a possible cause of anemia. *Assessment/Physiologic Integrity (Rosdahl, 1995, p. 218)*

10. **(B)** Correct. The length of the urethra is much shorter in the female and, because of this, bacteria that enters the urethra has a shorter distance to travel to enter the bladder. Hence, this is one reason that females have a higher incidence of UTIs than their male counterparts. (A), (C), and (D) Incorrect. These are not the reasons that women have a greater incidence of UTIs than men. *Data Collection/Health Promotion (Thompson, McFarland, Hirsch, and Tucker, 1997, p. 995)*

11. **(A)** Correct. This soft tissue edema can occur as a result of the trauma of delivery. (B) Incorrect. This is a result of bleeding in the subperiosteal area and does not cross suture lines. (C) Incorrect. This is a rash that will go away soon after birth and has no pathologic significance. (D) Incorrect. This is considered abnormal and can represent increased intracranial pressure. *Data Collection/Physiologic Integrity (Sherwen, Scoloveno, and Weingarten, 1991, p. 751)*

12. **(B)** Correct. Tingling and numbness could represent nerve damage and a decreased amount of blood circulating in the area. Perfusion assessment in the area beyond the cast is essential, and these complaints warrant immediate attention. (A), (C), and (D) Incorrect. All of these conditions would require additional assessment and reporting but are not an immediate, life-threatening concern. *Evaluation/Physiologic Integrity (Ellis, Nowlis, and Bentz, 1996, p. 557)*

13. **(A)** Correct. Just as in CPR, the first and foremost concern is the airway and ability to breathe. Without this, all other functions will cease quickly. (B), (C), and (D) Incorrect. These are all important but are related, directly or indirectly, to circulation and have a lower priority than airway maintenance. *Data Collection/Physiologic Integrity (Scherer and Timby, 1995, p. 234)*

14. **(C)** Correct. The urinary catheter should be clamped off for short periods of time only, in order to obtain a small sample of urine. Longer periods of time may cause the urine to back up into the bladder and increase the potential for UTIs. (A), (B), and (D) Incorrect. These times are either too short or too long for collection to take place. *Implementation/Physiologic Integrity (Christensen and Kockrow, 1995, p. 317)*

15. **(B)** Correct. This break in confidentiality of client information requires immediate intervention. The nurse must address the problem immediately. (A) Incorrect. This may be done later but the initial priority is to discontinue the breach of confidentiality. (C) Incorrect. The nursing assistants must be spoken to at once; after the meal would be too late to stop this particular incident. (D) Incorrect. The responsibility of the nurse is to stop the breach and inform their supervisor. Others will consider the need to discuss this with the client's family or not. *Evaluation/Safe Environment (Rosdahl, 1995, p. 34)*

16. **(A)** Correct. This medication acts as a paste covering the ulcer. The best time to give this medication is just prior to eating so it will protect the ulceration from the increase in hydrochloric acid being secreted during mealtime. (B) Incorrect. If administered at this time, it will be too late to work appropriately. (C) and (D) Incorrect. These times of administration are inappropriate. *Planning/Physiologic Integrity (Rosdahl, 1995, p. 711)*

17. **(B)** Correct. The addition of food coloring to the feeding solution will help uncover obvious and hidden aspiration. If the client is aspirating tube feedings and food color has been added,

then when the sputum secretions are suctioned from the lungs, the color will be similar to the food coloring added. (A), (C), and (D) Incorrect. None of these will be of assistance in determining whether the client has aspirated feeding solution. *Evaluation/Physiologic Integrity (Ellis, Nowlis, and Bentz, 1996, p. 706)*

18. **(A)** Correct. During periods of exacerbation, or acute inflammation, active range of motion (especially to pain) can cause significant joint damage. Consequently, range of motion should be done by the nurse but not to pain or beyond. (B), (C), and (D) Incorrect. These are all appropriate measures to employ during the acute stage of the illness. *Planning/Physiologic Integrity (Ellis, Nowlis, and Bentz, 1996, p. 537)*

19. **(C)** Correct. Nitrates act directly on the smooth muscle of the coronary vessels to produce vasodilatation. They can also dilate other blood vessels as well and can cause a headache. Their primary use is in the relief of anginal attacks. (A) Incorrect. This medication does not usually cause a headache as a side effect. (B) Incorrect. Acetaminophen is not usually used to relieve cardiac pain of this type. (D) Incorrect. This medication is frequently used to manage the pain associated with myocardial infarction, although it may be used in severe forms of angina. It is not, however, the drug of choice and is usually given intravenously. *Implementation/Physiologic Integrity (Eckler and Fair, 1996, p. 286)*

20. **(C)** Correct. In order to ensure an accurate reading the scale must be balanced at zero. (A) Incorrect. The height is usually done after the weight. (B) Incorrect. Privacy should be provided to decrease client anxiety, but balancing the scale is done first. (D) Incorrect. The client should stand on the scale after it is balanced. *Implementation/Physiologic Integrity (Christensen and Kockrow, 1995, p. 164)*

21. **(A)** Correct. One side effect or expected change for a person taking Dilantin is that he or she will develop a pink-tinged urine. This is to be expected, and the parents and child should be informed of this. (B), (C), and (D) Incorrect. None of these findings are considered to be an expected result of taking this medication. *Evaluation/Physiologic Integrity (Wong, 1997, p. 1022)*

22. **(D)** Correct. The client is simply seeking information about what is going to happen during the interview and what to expect. While these types of interviews may be routine for the nurse, they are not for the client and may need additional clarification. (A) Incorrect. This is not true and is not the reason for the interview. (B) Incorrect. The client may or may not be concerned, but at this point, the conclusion cannot be drawn from his question. (C) Incorrect. This does not address the client's question. *Evaluation/Psychosocial Integrity (Bailey and Bailey, 1993, p. 130)*

23. **(B)** Correct. To maximize healing and relaxation, the sitz bath should last from 20 to 30 minutes. (A), (C), and (D) Incorrect. These are all appropriate measures to utilize when a client is taking a sitz bath. *Implementation/Physiologic Integrity (Christensen and Kockrow, 1995, p. 272)*

24. **(D)** Correct. The response to a traumatic event may result in a loss of a physical function such as blindness, deafness, or paraplegia. (A), (B), and (C) Incorrect. These defense mechanisms are not associated with the complaint described. *Data Collection/Psychosocial Integrity (Bailey and Bailey, 1993, p. 34)*

25. **(A)** Correct. Pulmonary edema is a diffuse extravascular accumulation of fluid in the small air sacs (alveoli) and bronchi, which is a medical emergency. (B) Incorrect. The client will develop tachypnea and tachycardia and become profusely diaphoretic. Managing the diaphoresis in the initial stage is not a priority. (C) Incorrect. Anxiety is a major component of this dis-

ease process, but lying flat will make the person more anxious. (D) Incorrect. The client's pulse rate should be evaluated at least every 5 minutes during the acute phase of the disorder. *Implementation/Physiologic Integrity (Thompson, McFarland, Hirsch, and Tucker, 1997, p. 181)*

26. **(C)** Correct. The need to encourage high-protein foods is essential for proper maintenance of skin. A lack of protein will lead to promotion of skin breakdown and a lack of healing ability. (A) Incorrect. The position should be changed at least every two hours. (B) Incorrect. The pressure areas should be massaged with each turn, at least every two hours. (D) Incorrect. The daily shower would not be recommended for a person of this age because it would tend to dry skin, leading to potential cracking and breaking. *Planning/Physiologic Integrity (Perry and Potter, 1994, p. 121)*

27. **(D)** Correct. Eating frequent small meals will help to decrease the emptying of gastric acid into the duodenum, which helps relieve the pain of the duodenal ulcer. (A), (B), and (C) Incorrect. These statements would indicate a lack of knowledge about the condition and are not directly related to duodenal ulcer management. *Evaluation/Health Promotion (Thompson, McFarland, Hirsch, and Tucker, 1997, p. 719)*

28. **(B)** Correct. The developmental stage is extremely important when developing plans and when considering the health needs of the individual client. (A), (C), and (D) Incorrect. These are all important but do not have the level of significance that item B does. *Planning/Psychosocial Integrity (Wold, 1993, p. 32)*

29. **(C)** Correct. The provision of finger foods or foods that can be eaten on the move are good choices for this client. (A) Incorrect. The client would not be able to sit and concentrate long enough to observe the nurse's dining actions. (B) Incorrect. This would be difficult to evaluate and not healthy. (D) Incorrect. The client would probably not be able to focus long enough to prepare or assist in preparing a meal. *Implementation/Psychocosocial (Bailey and Bailey, 1993, p. 269)*

30. **(B)** Correct. Serum and blood products are the major means of transmission of hepatitis B and can be minimized using universal precautions. (A), (C), and (D) Incorrect. These people are at greater risk for developing hepatitis A. *Evaluation/Health Promotion (Ellis, Nowlis, and Bentz, 1996, p. 22)*

31. **(B)** Correct. When the left side of the heart fails to pump efficiently, blood backs up into the pulmonary veins and lung tissues. (A) Incorrect. Right-sided failure usually results in peripheral edema. Blood accumulates in the great vessels and backs up in peripheral veins. Because it has nowhere else to go, the extra fluid enters the tissues. (C) Incorrect. Pneumonia is an acute illness caused by inflammation or infection of the lungs. Auscultation of the chest may reveal wheezing, crackles, or rattling sounds in the chest and throat. (D) Incorrect. Emphysema is a chronic lung disease with distention of the alveolar walls due to loss of elasticity. Assessment shows marked shortness of breath after minimal activity. *Data Collection/Physiologic Integrity (Scherer and Timby, 1995, pp. 341, 299, and 307)*

32. **(C)** Correct. The tonic phase of a seizure is characterized by a tensing of the muscles that will occur just prior to the clonic phase of a generalized seizure. (A) Incorrect. The ictal phase means the seizure phase and includes all portions of the seizure. (B) Incorrect. The clonic phase is the time when the client begins to have a rhythmic moving of the extremities and body as seen in clonus. (D) Incorrect. The onset of the seizure can include a variety of physi-

cal motions or movements and is not directly associated with the tonic phase of a seizure. *Data Collection/Physiologic Integrity (Christensen and Kockrow, 1995, p. 1117)*

33. **(C)** Correct. An understanding of what is going to happen during a procedure can take some of the mystery away and reduce the anxiety of the client. (A) Incorrect. This will not serve to decrease anxiety. (B) Incorrect. This provides some information, but not the type that will decrease anxiety. (D) Incorrect. The determination of the test may be a cause for increasing anxiety; hence, this is not as effective a measure as item C. *Implementation/Health Promotion (Kalman and Waughfield, 1993, p. 90)*

34. **(B)** Correct. Within 24 to 48 hours after surgery, acute pain begins to subside. Pain medications are subsequently adjusted to meet the client's needs. The nurse should evaluate those needs first. (A) Incorrect. Even if ordered, the nurse should evaluate the pain level first. (C) and (D) Incorrect. These may be appropriate after the pain has been evaluated. *Evaluation/Physiologic Integrity (Christensen and Kockrow, 1995, p. 489)*

35. **(C)** Correct. This response seeks to clarify the reasoning and thought processes that the client is experiencing. (A) Incorrect. This answer is not acceptable, as it may provide a mixed message about what is known and unknown in this disorder. (B) Incorrect. This response does not actually respond to the client's question. (D) Incorrect. This response may be needed after the reason the question was asked has been identified. *Implementation/Psychosocial Integrity (Bailey and Bailey, 1993, p. 130)*

36. **(B)** Correct. Coughing, deep breathing, and the use of incentive spirometry may lack effectiveness if the client is in too much pain or too anxious to perform it. Splinting of the chest with a pillow, for example, can assist in maximizing breathing. (A) Incorrect. Moving about is important to prevent DVT formation and to help improve breathing, but it is not as important as item B. (C) Incorrect. The family can be of greater assistance if they are also taught to encourage the client to breathe in the same manner. (D) Incorrect. Suction at the bedside would be important, but not as important as preventative measures such as item B. *Implementation/Physiologic Integrity (Rosdahl, 1995, p. 634)*

37. **(C)** Correct. By most definitions, the difference between acute and chronic pain is associated with a length of time longer than 5 to 6 or more months. (A) and (B) Incorrect. This time is too short. (D) Incorrect. This time is too long to be the beginning of chronic pain. *Planning/Physiologic Integrity (Scherer and Timby, 1995, p. 166)*

38. **(B)** Correct. This position would place the head down and the feet up. The client with COPD experiences a condition known as orthopnea, which is difficulty breathing in the lying position. (A), (C), and (D) Incorrect. These positions would not pose as great a problem as the Trendelenburg's position. *Evaluation/Health Promotion (Thompson, McFarland, Hirsch, and Tucker, 1997, p. 151)*

39. **(C)** Correct. The use of denial helps to deal with information that is too traumatic and troubling to cope with. It will decrease anxiety levels for a while. (A) Incorrect. Projection occurs when the person projects his or her thoughts or beliefs onto another person and attributes them to the other person. It is easier to say "That person hates me" than it is to say "I hate that person." (B) Incorrect. Repression is a defense mechanism that occurs in response to tremendously painful or traumatic experiences. (D) Incorrect. Fantasy is not an actual defense mechanism, but it can be used to create a world more acceptable and less threatening to the person. *Data Collection/Psychosocial Integrity (Bailey and Bailey, 1993, p. 33)*

40. **(C)** Correct. An increase in the pulse rate to 140 beats per minute indicates that the heart is not compensating for the increased energy demand as it should. The activity should be terminated. (A) Incorrect. Complaints of feeling tired and weak are frequently expressed by many postoperative clients when they resume walking. (B) Incorrect. Nausea may be a result of a number of problems including postoperative pain or lightheadedness, but neither is a complaint of the client. (D) Incorrect. A systolic blood pressure of 110 mm Hg is not unusual and would not be an indicator the client is not tolerating the procedure. *Evaluation/Physiologic Integrity (Scherer and Timby, 1995, p. 392)*

41. **(A)** Correct. A delusion is defined as a fixed, false belief. That means that it is difficult to reason with, because the individual has a fixed belief that defies description. (B) Incorrect. A hallucination is a sensory experience unique to that person. (C) Incorrect. An illusion is a misperception of reality. (D) Incorrect. This is not an example of symbolism. *Data Collection/Psychosocial Integrity (Bailey and Bailey, 1993, p. 248)*

42. **(D)** Correct. The wound needs to be covered immediately, and the covering should be dampened with a sterile solution. (A), (B), and (C) Incorrect. These are all important, but covering the wound is the first intervention that should be performed. *Implementation/Physiologic Integrity (Christensen and Kockrow, 1995, p. 454)*

43. **(A)** Correct. This would indicate that the client may be having a major problem that is creating a shock-like response. This requires immediate notification of the charge nurse. (B) Incorrect. The condition is not known and does not have the greatest priority. (C) Incorrect. This is not an acceptable answer. Licensed practical/vocational nurses do not initiate oxygen therapy without a physician's order. (D) Incorrect. This is not an intervention that would be performed at this time with this client. *Planning/Physiologic Integrity (Wong, 1997, p. 896)*

44. **(A)** Correct. A rise in the pulse rate is one of the earliest signs of shock. (B) Incorrect. This is considered a normal blood pressure and does not reflect shock. (C) Incorrect. A respiratory range of 24 falls into the normal range, although it is on the high normal side. (D) Incorrect. The temperature of 101°F is not associated directly with a sign of shock but can indicate many other problems. *Data Collection/Physiologic Integrity (Scherer and Timby, 1995, p. 207)*

45. **(C)** Correct. Whenever the nurse cannot identify a person without a name band, he or she should always ask the person who he is rather than stating his name. (A) Incorrect. The client's roommate may not be a reliable person. (B) Incorrect. Other staff who are familiar with the resident can help as well, but they may not know the client either. This is why identification bands are essential in safe practice. (D) Incorrect. Checking the client's record may be a safe alternative, but only if it contains a recent picture of the client. *Implementation/Safe Environment (Wold, 1993, p. 338)*

46. **(B)** Correct. When providing nutrition, the first thing the nurse should ensure is that the correct person is getting the correct tray. Otherwise, dangerous accidents could occur with diabetic clients or clients on MAO inhibitors, for example. (A) Incorrect. The foods the client requested may not be the foods he can eat on the specific diet he is on. (C) Incorrect. The proper diet for the client is very important, but it is essential that the correct client receives the correct meal. This would be the second step. (D) Incorrect. A comfortable, safe eating position is important, but item B has greater priority and is of highest import. *Planning/ Safe Environment (Ellis, Nowlis, and Bentz, 1996, p. 362)*

47. (A) Correct. If the suction is not operating with a sucking capacity that would be expected, the suction may not be properly turned on, or the connections may be inadequate and the pressure may be leaking. (B) and (C) Incorrect. Troubleshooting by the nurse should be performed prior to notifying the supervisor or the plant manager. (D) Incorrect. This may need to be done, but only after item A has been performed. *Implementation/Safe Environment (Thompson, McFarland, Hirsch, and Tucker, 1997, p. 197)*

48. (D) Correct. Shearing force is the friction created by moving a client over a surface. This type of force can cause skin damage and be the first step in creating a pressure sore. It will create an opening in the skin in that organisms can enter, thus breaking the protective barrier. (A) Incorrect. Proper positioning and range of motion will help to prevent contractures, but this is not a major consideration when turning a client. (B) Incorrect. Soiling the linen would not be a major consideration when moving or turning a client. It would be important for the nurse to make sure the linen was not soiled prior to turning the client. (C) Incorrect. Changing the pull sheet with every turn is not necessary. *Planning/Physiologic Integrity (Ellis, Nowlis, and Bentz, 1996, p. 334)*

49. (A) Correct. This item is a direct action and is considered a nursing intervention by all definitions. (B), (C), and (D) Incorrect. These items are all considered part of data collection and are not considered to be nursing interventions. *Implementation/Physiologic Integrity (Ellis, Nowlis, and Bentz, 1996, p. 11)*

50. (D) Correct. The skin of the aging client is not able to replace oils as rapidly as younger individuals; therefore, it would be of greater benefit for an older client to have less frequent complete baths and partial baths on alternate days. (A), (B), and (C) Incorrect. All of these clients could benefit from a daily bath, and it would not be contraindicated. *Planning/Health Promotion (Ellis, Nowlis, and Bentz, 1996, p. 410)*

51. (C) Correct. When establishing baseline and changes in weights, the most important consideration is consistency. This requires that the person be weighed at the same time every day. (A) Incorrect. The nurse would want to know the weight of the client before diuretics are administered so that the amount of fluid lost after introduction of the diuretic can be evaluated by comparing pre- and postdiuretic weights. (B) Incorrect. The clothing that the client wears is a consideration, and individual institutions have policies about this. (D) Incorrect. The meals may have little impact on any given weight. *Planning/Health Promotion (Rosdahl, 1995, p. 447)*

52. (B) Correct. The amount of fluid retained can be determined by the weight gain. The accepted ratio, one liter, is equivalent to one kilogram or 2.2 pounds. This client had gained $4\frac{1}{2}$ pounds, or roughly two liters of fluid. (A), (C), and (D) Incorrect. None of these is considered a correct relationship to the amount of fluid retained. *Evaluation/Physiologic Integrity (Thompson, McFarland, Hirsch, and Tucker, 1997, p. 1556)*

53. (D) Correct. The treatment can cause a temporary confusional state which will resolve within several hours after treatment. This is the reason that most decisions regarding aftercare are developed prior to the treatment. (A) Incorrect. Depression may still continue and usually requires a course of treatments to resolve. (B) Incorrect. The person should not be left alone immediately after the treatment and should be closely monitored for potential airway and breathing difficulties. (C) Incorrect. Urinary incontinence can be controlled by having the client void in advance of the procedure; fecal incontinence is a rare occurrence. *Planning/Psychosocial Integrity (Bailey and Bailey, 1993, p. 170)*

54. (B) Correct. This complaint may indicate that the water is too cold and is causing unnecessary body temperature changes. (A) Incorrect. The sitz bath is used to relieve perineal discomfort; this should help to decrease it. (C) Incorrect. There is no relationship between sitz baths and constipation. (D) Incorrect. This may occur when using a sitz bath but would be an expected comment that would not require any intervention. *Evaluation/Physiologic Integrity (Rosdahl, 1995, p. 574)*

55. (C) Correct. It is important to make sure the wheelchair is on the client's "good" or unaffected side so that when she transfers to it, she will be able to use her strong side to assist in the transfer. (A) Incorrect. This could place the wheelchair to the client's affected side and would make transfers more dangerous. (B) Incorrect. This wheelchair position would require the client to make a 180-degree turn to transfer. (D) Incorrect. This would not be an appropriate angle for the wheelchair to be located in a transfer. *Planning/Physiologic Integrity (Ellis, Nowlis, and Bentz, 1996, p. 462)*

56. (A) Correct. The sigmoid colon and descending colon are located in the left lower quadrant of the abdomen, and placing the client on the left side allows gravity to assist in the flowing and retention of the fluid instilled via enema. (B) and (D) Incorrect. A semirecumbent position will make it difficult to perform the procedure and will make it difficult to retain the fluid for any length of time. (C) Incorrect. This position would be contraindicated because gravity would be working against the instillation of the solution, making retention very difficult. *Implementation/Safe Environment (Ellis, Nowlis, and Bentz, 1996, p. 686)*

57. (C) Correct. The foot size is not a needed measurement for proper fitting of antithrombotic stockings. (A), (B), and (D) Incorrect. All of these measurements are needed in order to properly fit the client with antithrombotic stockings. *Implementation/Physiologic Integrity (Ellis, Nowlis, and Bentz, 1996, p. 628)*

58. (C) Correct. By encouraging the mother to participate and hold the client, the nurse can provide comfort to both the client and mother and can give the mother something meaningful to do. (A) Incorrect. This would be done but is not the most appropriate selection. (B) Incorrect. The client would not necessarily be medicated after a blood test. (D) Incorrect. This response would not be as appropriate in light of first having her mother hold her. *Implementation/Psychosocial Integrity (Wong, 1997, pp. 832, 883)*

59. (C) Correct. This temperature is high enough not to cause "gooseflesh," which could increase shivering and a fever, yet low enough not to encourage hyperthermia, or increased body temperature. (A), (B), and (D) Incorrect. None of these temperatures are considered correct when performing a tepid sponge bath. *Planning/Physiologic Integrity (Rosdahl, 1995, p. 574)*

60. (B) Correct. An unretracted foreskin can act as a tourniquet over the end of the penis and can cut off circulation and create swelling and edema. (A) Incorrect. There is no association between erection response and an unretracted foreskin. (C) Incorrect. Urinary tract infection potential is decreased with proper perineal care. (D) Incorrect. While perineal care itself may prove to be embarrassing to the client, it is not related to the reason the foreskin must be retracted. *Implementation/Physiologic Integrity (Rosdahl, 1995, p. 523)*

61. (C) Correct. One significant way to assist the confused person to orient himself to place is by placing his name in areas of importance, such as on the doorway to his room, near his bed and on his dressers and bureaus. (A) Incorrect. This does not help him understand where he is, only where he is not. (B) Incorrect. Group therapy that may be of help to him is reality orientation, but most confused individuals do not respond to group therapy because the confusion also often creates an attention deficit as well. (D) Incorrect. This action will confuse the person even more, as the coming and going of different staff members can increase his confusional state. *Implementation/Psychosocial Integrity (Wold, 1993, p. 263)*

62. **(B)** Correct. Clients who are experiencing nephrotic syndrome or renal failure should have all sources of potassium restricted, as hyperkalemia will cause dangerous cardiac irregularities that would threaten the client's life. (A), (C), and (D) Incorrect. These fruits can be used in moderation in this client. *Planning/Physiologic Integrity (Wong, 1997, p. 972)*

63. **(B)** Correct. The proper method for opening and creating a sterile field is to open the first fold away from the body. This will prevent the need to reach across the sterile area when opening the other folds, or when placing objects on the field. (A), (C), and (D) Incorrect. These may cause an inadvertent contamination of the field. *Implementation/Safe Environment (Rosdahl, 1995, p. 642)*

64. **(D)** Correct. The normal top portion of the abdominal binder should be below the costal margins, as this will not affect respiratory capacity or the ribs from moving with respiration or breathing. (A) and (B) Incorrect. The level of this binder placement is too high and may affect respirations. (C) Incorrect. This is too low and would not provide the necessary support. *Implementation/Physiologic Integrity (Ellis, Nowlis, and Bentz, 1996, p. 623)*

65. **(B)** Correct. It is important that the client remain very still during this procedure, and the nurse must intervene to ensure safety. This means making sure the client remains in the proper position. (A) Incorrect. This is not necessary. (C) Incorrect. This is not a painless procedure and to assure the client's family of this would be misinforming them. (D) Incorrect. The vital signs would be measured pre- and postprocedure, but obtaining them during the procedure would be extremely difficult and impractical. *Planning/Physiologic Integrity (Wong, 1997, p. 706)*

66. **(D)** Correct. When obtaining a 24-hour composite urine sample, the client should be encouraged to void one last time at the conclusion of the test, even if they recently voided. (A) Incorrect. Fluid intake is always important when considering urinary output but is not a specific requirement for this test. (B) Incorrect. The client does not need an indwelling Foley catheter for this test. (C) Incorrect. This is not necessary and is not a concern in this type of test. *Implementation/Health Promotion (Rosdahl, 1995, p. 556)*

67. **(D)** Correct. A respiratory rate of 36 falls out of all parameters of normalcy and should be reported immediately. (A) Incorrect. This blood pressure is slightly elevated and should be rechecked first. (B) Incorrect. This pulse rate is only slightly elevated and should be rechecked first. (C) Incorrect. This slight temperature elevation should be reported, but it does not have the immediacy of a respiratory rate of 36. *Data Collection/Physiologic Integrity (Ellis, Nowlis, and Bentz, 1996, p. 133)*

68. **(D)** Correct. After a cast has been placed, it is essential to monitor the extremity for any signs of neurovascular complications. (A) Incorrect. This may be important in some specific situations but is not the highest priority in this. (B) Incorrect. This is an important part of care of the cast client, but it is not the highest priority. (C) Incorrect. Assessing for pain is important, but this is done prior to application of the cast and is not as high a priority. *Evaluation/Physiologic Integrity (Ellis, Nowlis, and Bentz, 1996, p. 570)*

69. **(D)** Correct. A urine collection for sugar and ketones should be recent. If the bladder has been collecting urine all night, then the information obtained in this specimen does not identify the current glucose and ketone state. (A) Incorrect. Sterility is not necessary for this test. (B) Incorrect. The test should be performed after obtaining the specimen. (C) Incorrect. A clean catch collection is not necessary. *Planning/Health Promotion (Ellis, Nowlis, and Bentz, 1996, p. 225)*

70. **(D)** Correct. Normal urine specific gravity ranges from 1.005 to 1.025. This low specific gravity would indicate an inability to concentrate the urine and could be reflective of a condition such as diabetes insipidus. (A), (B), and (C) Incorrect. These are all expected findings in a urine specimen. *Data Collection/Physiologic Integrity (Ellis, Nowlis, and Bentz, 1996, p. 223)*

71. **(C)** Correct. The cold pack should be applied at least several times per day; a once-a-day application will serve to do little in the recovery process. (A), (B), and (D) Incorrect. These are all appropriate interventions and indicate correct understanding of care of the sprain. *Evaluation/Health Promotion (Rosdahl, 1995, p. 1007)*

72. **(B)** Correct. The auditory hallucination is the most frequently occurring type of hallucination. (A), (C), and (D) Incorrect. These can also occur with schizophrenia but are less frequently observed. *Data Collection/Psychosocial Integrity (Bailey and Bailey, 1993, p. 248)*

73. **(D)** Correct. Liquid ferrous sulfate will stain the teeth; therefore, drinking it with a straw is mandatory. (A) and (B) Incorrect. This medication should not be mixed with any other type of flavoring that will inhibit absorption. (C) Incorrect. This should never be a consideration in taking medication. This recommendation can prove dangerous to children, as they may take medication under the belief they are taking more candy. *Implementation/Physiologic Integrity (Wong, 1997, p. 910)*

74. **(B)** Correct. A kyphotic curve is one that makes the client appear hunched over and is seen in many elderly individuals, especially those suffering from severe osteoporosis and thinning of the cervical disks. (A) Incorrect. This is known as lordosis. (C) Incorrect. The lateral deviation of the spine is known as scoliosis. (D) Incorrect. This may have an impact on the neck because these are neck muscles, but it is not directly associated with kyphosis. *Data Collection/Physiologic Integrity (Rosdahl, 1995, p. 180)*

75. **(A)** Correct. Placement of the chair at the head of the bed and facing down toward the client's feet is a good position for the client to transfer to and to sit in to observe the activities within the room. (B), (C), and (D) Incorrect. All of these positions will decrease sensory stimulation or make it more difficult to transfer into the chair. *Planning/Physiologic Integrity (Ellis, Nowlis, and Bentz, 1996, p. 462)*

76. **(C)** Correct. Standing closer than one arm's length away can create anxiety in people, as it invades their personal space. The general rule in working in the mental health area is to remain at least at this distance. (A) Incorrect. There is no indication of a sexual attraction in the situation. (B) Incorrect. This may be part of why anyone feels uncomfortable during the invasion of personal space, but it is not the main reason. (D) Incorrect. No evidence exists that would support this answer. *Evaluation/Psychosocial Integrity (Bailey and Bailey, 1993, p. 126)*

77. **(B)** Correct. The use of respiratory precautions, especially using a special mask with a filter, is indicated, along with the use of gloves as indicated by universal precaution procedures. (A), (C), and (D) Incorrect. A gown is not indicated in managing a pulmonary tuberculosis client. *Planning/Safe Environment (Rosdahl, 1995, p. 1197)*

78. **(B)** Correct. The first intervention performed in any environmental accident is to remove all people who may be at risk for injury. Many institutions use the mnemonic device of RACE for their fire-fighting policy: R for remove, A for alarm, C for contain, and E for extinguish. (A), (C), and (D) Incorrect. All of the other options have a lower priority than removing the clients from immediate harm. *Implementation/Safe Environment (Christensen and Kockrow, 1995, p. 219)*

79. **(A)** Correct. This information represents that obtained in the past health history. (B) Incorrect. This information is obtained in the family history. (C) Incorrect. This occupational information is part of the social history. (D) Incorrect. This education information is part of the social history. *Data Collection/Health Promotion (Rosdahl, 1995, p. 384)*

80. **(B)** Correct. A high-residue diet is recommended for a person who is suffering from constipation. A low-residue diet will create more constipation and is the diet of choice in diseases such as ulcerative colitis. (A), (C), and (D) Incorrect. These are all answers that indicate a knowledge of how to prevent constipation. *Evaluation/Health Promotion (Wold, 1993, p. 202)*

81. **(B)** Correct. The therapeutic intervention is to stay with the client for a selected period of time. By allowing this, the nurse is telling the client that she is important to her and that it is all right to talk or not talk, whichever she prefers. (A) Incorrect. This is the wrong reason to stay with a client and would not be a therapeutic response. (C) Incorrect. This is a generalization and is too superficial a response. (D) Incorrect. The use of "why" in a response is not considered an appropriate intervention because it makes the person being questioned defensive. *Planning/Psychosocial Integrity (Bailey and Bailey, 1993, p. 129)*

82. **(C)** Correct. The type that would be more likely to have a need for irrigation is the sigmoid colostomy, as the stool appears similar in consistency to normal stool. (A), (B), and (D) Incorrect. These are less likely to have a need for irrigation. *Implementation/Physiologic Integrity (Scherer and Timby, 1995, p. 731)*

83. **(B)** Correct. Use of a lancet on the tip or pad of the finger is an improper method of obtaining a blood sample. It is extremely painful and is a reason for noncompliance with the testing process. The side of the finger should be used to pierce. (A), (C), and (D) Incorrect. These are all proper methods for obtaining an accurate blood glucose and should be taught. *Evaluation/Physiologic Integrity (Ellis, Nowlis, and Bentz, 1996, p. 243)*

84. **(B)** Correct. This is the standard for assessing for compete pulselessness and complete respiratory arrest. (A), (C), and (D) Incorrect. These are either too short a period or too long a period. *Data Collection/Physiologic Integrity (Ellis, Nowlis, and Bentz, 1996, p. 725)*

85. **(B)** Correct. The charge nurse is the first person to speak to and should be notified immediately in the event of a medication error. (A) Incorrect. Informing the client may cause undue panic if the error did not actually occur. He or she may be informed at some point during the process, but not necessarily immediately. (C) Incorrect. The physician will need to be informed, but this usually occurs after the charge nurse has been notified and collected detailed information from the medication nurse. (D) Incorrect. As part of the evaluation of the error, the order would be checked again, but usually after the charge nurse has been notified. *Evaluation/Health Promotion (Rosdahl, 1995, p. 716)*

86. **(D)** Correct. The client who has memory deficits will lose his own identity last when the confusional state is progressing. The day, time, and year may be lost in any client who has been hospitalized or institutionalized for any length of time. (A) Incorrect. He may not realistically

know where he is. (B) Incorrect. The date and year may become lost over time in long-term hospitalization. (C) Incorrect. The time of day may not be known unless it has direct significance for the person being asked. Clients in intensive care units may lose track of time and not know day from night. *Evaluation/Psychosocial Integrity (Bailey and Bailey, 1997, p. 133)*

87. **(B)** Correct. Streptococcal infections that remain untreated can end up infecting the heart, the heart valves, and the kidneys, causing kidney failure or nephrotic syndrome. (A), (C), and (D) Incorrect. These conditions may be associated with septic infections, but they are not as predominant as kidney disease. *Planning/Physiologic Integrity (Wong, 1997, p. 966)*

88. **(B)** Correct. Manic clients are very impulsive and unpredictable. As a consequence, they are at risk for injury to themselves and others. (A) Incorrect. The inclusion of manic clients in any type of group activities such as this is not recommended, as they are too impulsive and disruptive. (C) Incorrect. This may be true in the person during a depressive episode of the bipolar disorder, but it is not a general rule. (D) Incorrect. Sexual promiscuity may be a problem, but polyphagia is not a usual problem with manic clients, as they don't concentrate long enough to have an appetite. *Planning/Psychosocial Integrity (Bailey and Bailey, 1993, p. 81)*

89. **(A)** Correct. The nasal cannula is the delivery system of choice for all clients who are receiving low-flow oxygen. This allows them to breathe, talk, and eat without interrupting the oxygen flow. (B) Incorrect. The simple face mask is the choice in emergency situations. (C) Incorrect. A Venturi mask delivers a very accurate flow rate of oxygen. (D) Incorrect. A nonrebreathing mask is used to provide 100 percent oxygen. *Implementation/Physiologic Integrity (Christensen and Kockrow, 1995, p. 924)*

90. **(A)** Correct. The wheelchair should be positioned so that the client's strong side is able to be fully utilized. (B) Incorrect. The nurse should instruct the nursing assistant in the proper method of transferring this client. (C) and (D) Incorrect. Neither of these responses would be appropriate. *Evaluation/Physiologic Integrity (Ellis, Nowlis, and Bentz, 1996, p. 462)*

91. **(B)** Correct. Stimulating the anal reflex prior to insertion of any object will cause an initial anal contraction and then a relaxation. The relaxation response is the time when the insertion should occur. (A) Incorrect. The client should be encouraged to relax just prior to inserting the suppository. (C) Incorrect. Taking a deep breath is acceptable, but the client should not be instructed to hold his breath, as it may cause more of a pressure or resistance to the insertion. (D) Incorrect. This procedure may increase the resistance to insertion of a suppository and would not be recommended. *Implementation/Physiologic Integrity (Christensen and Kockrow, 1995, p. 411)*

92. **(A)** Correct. Urinary retention is a problem that requires immediate attention and can be considered a medical emergency, as the inability to void may create additional renal disorders such as hydronephrosis. (B) Incorrect. This disorder is associated with inflammation or infection and is not as pressing a problem as lack of urine. (C) and (D) Incorrect. These are signs of enlarged prostate or early partial obstruction. *Data Collection/Physiologic Integrity (Thompson, McFarland, Hirsch, and Tucker, 1997, p. 1033)*

93. **(D)** Correct. This is not considered a sign of hypoglycemia; rather, it is associated with ketoacidosis and elevated blood sugars. In hypoglycemia the skin becomes pale, moist, and cool. (A), (B) and (C) Incorrect. These all would be included in the teaching of how to avoid hypoglycemia. *Planning/Physiologic Integrity (Scherer and Timby, 1995, p. 806)*

94. **(D)** Correct. Subjective data is considered information that the client reports. (A), (B), and (C) Incorrect. These are not considered to be subjective information. *Data Collection/Physiologic Integrity (Perry and Potter, 1994, p. 31)*

95. **(D)** Correct. The best method for reducing or preventing nipple soreness is to properly place and encourage the infant to take in the entire areola. (A) Incorrect. This may be a recommendation if the nipples become very painful but would not be a nursing action. (B) Incorrect. Lanolin or a wet tea bag could be applied to the nipple, but lotion is not recommended. (C) Incorrect. The increased tension and improper removal from the breast can cause more nipple soreness. *Implementation/Health Promotion (Sherwen, Scoloveno, and Weingarten, 1991, p. 673)*

96. **(A)** Correct. The correct steps to assure placement would be to (1) aspirate GI contents with a syringe; (2) auscultate with a stethoscope over the left upper quadrant of the abdomen and rapidly inject 10 to 20 mL of air without resistance via syringe into a tube. (B) Incorrect. Flushing the tube with water without checking placement may create aspiration. (C) Incorrect. This would be done after the tube has been aspirated. (D) Incorrect. This would not check tube placement. *Implementation/Physiologic Integrity (Perry and Potter, 1994, p. 700)*

97. **(B)** Correct. Clients with Crohn's disease complain of diarrhea of three to six semisolid stools daily containing mucus and pus but no blood. Intestinal fistulas or poor absorption of bile salts may cause stools to be watery. (A) Incorrect. Rectal bleeding and abdominal cramping are signs of ulcerative colitis. (C) Incorrect. Right lower abdominal pain with rebound tenderness are signs of appendicitis. (D) Incorrect. Gastroesophageal reflux is a sign of hiatal hernia or an esophageal problem. *Data Collection/Physiologic Integrity (Thompson, McFarland, Hirsch, and Tucker, 1997, p. 751)*

98. **(C)** Correct. This medication, known as Pepto-Bismol, is used for upset stomach, diarrhea, and as part of the treatment for peptic ulcer disease due to *Helicobacter pylori*. (A), (B), and (D) Incorrect. All have a main action associated with the antacids. *Implementation/Physiologic Integrity (Eckler and Fair, 1996, p. 367)*

99. **(C)** Correct. Dysphasia, or difficult swallowing, would be the most important presenting symptom, along with the sensation of food being stuck in her throat. (A) Incorrect. Constipation would not be a symptom on initial assessment. (B) Incorrect. Hematemesis may be presenting symptom for an esophageal or peptic ulcer. (D) Incorrect. Hoarseness would more likely be associated with laryngeal cancer. *Data Collection/Physiologic Integrity (Christensen and Kockrow, 1995, p. 663)*

100. **(D)** Correct. The surgical intervention that involves creating a small bladder with a portion of the ileum and a valve on the surface of the skin is known as Kock's pouch. The client will not have any need for large external appliances after this procedure. (A), (B), and (C) Incorrect. All of these procedures will result in a need for an external collection bag. *Implementation/Physiologic Integrity (Scherer and Timby, 1995, p. 951)*

101. **(C)** Correct. This is the proper depth of compressions as recommended by the American Heart Association and the American Red Cross. (A), (B), and (D) Incorrect. These do not fit the recommendations for depth of compressions in the adult. *Implementation/Physiologic Integrity (Ellis, Nowlis, and Bentz, 1996, p. 726)*

102. (B) Correct. This is considered a probable sign of pregnancy and occurs when the mucous membranes of the genitalia and cervix take on a bluish color. (A), (C), and (D) Incorrect. These would not be an accurate description of Chadwick's sign. *Data Collection/Health Promotion (Sherwen, Scoloveno, and Weingarten, 1991, p. 305)*

103. (A) Correct. It is a nursing responsibility to ensure that the client remains safe. Contamination of a sterile field can lead to infections and an increased infection risk. (B) Incorrect. If a sterile field has been compromised, there are no portions that can be used. (C) Incorrect. A need to obtain another sterile field should be part of the reason for going to get another one. The nurse setting up the field should be informed of how she contaminated the field. (D) Incorrect. If the contaminated field is used, client safety has been jeopardized. *Evaluation/Implementation (Rosdahl, 1995, p. 642)*

104. (C) Correct. Not covering the skin is an important intervention because additional damage to the skin can occur if it is exposed to a moist environment for a prolonged period. (A), (B), and (D) Incorrect. These are not considered effective methods for the correct use of a wet-to-dry dressing. *Implementation/Physiologic Integrity (Christensen and Kockrow, 1995, p. 470)*

105. (D) Correct. The need for assessment of the reason for this confusion is paramount at this point and should be evaluated as soon as possible. (A) Incorrect. Administration of this medication at this time may mask the underlying problem. (B) Incorrect. This would be difficult and would not be appropriate at this point. (C) Incorrect. Notifying her family would not solve the problem and would only create more problems for the family without addressing the client's problem. *Implementation/Psychosocial Integrity (Bailey and Bailey, 1993, p. 259)*

106. (A) Correct. This type of seizure is one that can be mistaken for daydreaming. In children, it may be discovered in school when the child is not able to answer questions posed by the teacher or is thought to be inattentive. (B) Incorrect. This type of seizure has a motor component but can also be mistaken for fainting or passing out. (C) Incorrect. This is the characteristic associated with a generalized or grand mal seizure. (D) Incorrect. This is a motor seizure and is not part of the absence seizure. *Data Collection/Physiologic Integrity (Christensen and Kockrow, 1995, p. 117)*

107. (D) Correct. When performing a CT scan, the client will be asked to lie very still. Movement during the procedure will render the test useless. (A), (B), and (C) Incorrect. All of these statements indicate an understanding of the test. *Evaluation/Health Promotion (Scherer and Timby, 1995, p. 149)*

108. (C) Correct. Whenever a person has difficulty breathing, sitting him up will usually assist in improving his breathing ability. (A), (B), and (D) Incorrect. These will not have the same effectiveness as sitting the client up. *Implementation/Physiologic Integrity (Ellis, Nowlis, and Bentz, 1996, p. 339)*

109. (D) Correct. Needlessly uncovering the client during a bath provides a means by which they may be exposed to a hypothermic state, may cause shivering and an increase in body temperature, and expose them or others to embarrassment. It should be addressed by the nurse immediately. (A, (B), and (C) Incorrect. This situation needs immediate attention and should be addressed at that time. *Evaluation/Physiologic Integrity (Rosdahl, 1995, p. 524)*

110. (B) Correct. Actelectasis is a condition in which the small air sacs, the alveoli, collapse due to lack of air. In order to prevent this, clients need to make a special effort to breathe deeply to ventilate all the alveoli in the bases of their lungs. This condition can lead to pneumonia. (A) Incorrect. Pulmonary edema occurs as a result of congestive heart failure. (C) Incorrect. Pneumothorax is a condition in which a lung, or a portion of a lung, collapses. (D) Incorrect. Pulmonary embolism is a potential complication in the postoperative recovery period, but this occurs as a result of development of a deep vein thrombosis (DVT). *Implementation/Physiologic Integrity (Christensen and Kockrow, 1995, p. 455)*

111. **(B)** Correct. This may indicate that the client is suffering from a ketoacidosis state and requires immediate intervention. (A) Incorrect. A complaint of decreased appetite may require an adjustment of insulin, but is not as an immediate concern as B. (C) Incorrect. Urinary output would be increased in hyperglycemia. (D) Incorrect. A craving for sweets would not necessarily require immediate attention. *Data Collection/Physiologic Integrity (Thompson, McFarland, Hirsch, and Tucker, 1997, p. 844)*

112. **(B)** Correct. Persons with decreased immune system are subject to fungal or candidal infections. Infection of the mouth is known as "thrush" and is treated with antifungals. (A), (C), and (D) Incorrect. These conditions are considered part of a profound immune system failure and are not commonly associated with the immune system of a newborn. *Data Collection/Physiologic Integrity (Wong, 1997, p. 225)*

113. **(C)** Correct. Hypovolemic shock is associated with fluid or blood loss. Hypotension would be the earliest sign of these four possibilities. (A), (B), and (D) Incorrect. These can occur in shock, but would occur later than hypotension. Bradycardia would occur only at the very end of life. *Data Collection/Physiologic Integrity (Scherer and Timby, 1995, p. 209)*

114. **(D)** Correct. Skim milk is rich in vitamin D and calcium but not potassium. (A), (B), and (C) Incorrect. These foods all are rich in potassium. *Implementation/Physiologic Integrity (Scherer and Timby, 1995, p. 424)*

115. **(C)** Correct. This would prevent further entries from being entered at a later time. (A) Incorrect. All charting should be done as soon as possible following the care given to a client. No room should be left for later recording of information. (B) Incorrect. It would be unnecessary to do this if you drew a line from the previous entry. (D) Incorrect. This would be destroying part of a legal document, which of course, you would never do. *Data Collection/Safe Environment (Perry and Potter, 1994, p. 29)*

116. **(D)** Correct. Placing the patient in a sitting position when she is experiencing an inflammation of the pericardial sac of the heart will help to relieve some of the discomfort and facilitate breathing. (A), (B), and (C) Incorrect. These positions are less effective than when sitting upright. *Implementation/Physiologic Integrity (Christensen and Kockrow, 1994, p. 739)*

117. **(A)** Correct. The nurse should further define the extent of his disorientation and check how easily he can be reoriented. (B), (C), and (D) Incorrect. These interventions may be appropriate at later times, but the initial action should be to further assess this confusion. *Data Collection/Physiologic Integrity (Christensen and Kockrow, 1995, p. 1278)*

118. **(D)** Correct. This is the first step in the Heimlich maneuver and is employed while the person is still conscious. (A) Incorrect. The nurse has already done this. (B) Incorrect. This would be done after he has lost consciousness. (C) Incorrect. This is recommended for infants under one year of age. *Planning/Physiologic Integrity (Scherer and Timby, 1995, p. 251)*

119. **(C)** Correct. The proper use of pain medication is taught to include identifying when the pain begins and not waiting until the pain becomes severe or intolerable. If this occurs, a greater amount of pain medication may be required. (A) Incorrect. By the time this occurs, the pain medication may not be effective. (B) Incorrect. The recommendation by many health care professionals is to medicate the client for pain before activities that cause pain are begun. (D) Incorrect. This may be a recommendation for some types of pain, such as the pain associated with chronic arthritis, but is not recommended in most acute conditions. *Evaluation/Health Promotion (Rosdahl, 1995, p. 613)*

120. **(B)** Correct. If the tube were blocked somehow, then air would not be able to be introduced. This is an indication that the tube is not functional. (A) Incorrect. The amount of stomach contents would not indicate a problem with the tube patency unless no contents could be aspirated. (C) Incorrect. Blood coming from the tube opening would indicate a number of problems, but is not indicative of a patency problem. (D) Incorrect. This may indicate a problem with the gallbladder or possible obstruction in the GI tract, but if it could be aspirated, then it would not indicate a problem with the patency of the tube itself. *Evaluation/Physiologic Integrity (Christensen and Kockrow, 1995, p. 675)*

121. **(A)** Correct. Keeping the tubing below the level of the bladder and urethra will prevent backflow of urine into the urinary bladder. This will help to minimize UTIs. (B) and (C) Incorrect. These both may be done as long as the nurse follows the principle described in the correct answer. (D) Incorrect. If the client walks while holding the drainage bag, he or she must be taught to keep it below the level of the bladder and urethra. *Implementation/Physiologic Integrity (Christensen and Kockrow, 1995, p. 834)*

122. **(B)** Correct. The client who has a pacemaker in place should not have this test, as it could interrupt the electrical conductivity settings of the pacemaker, and the pacemaker or the pacemaker wires could become accidentally moved or dislodged. (A) Incorrect. This is not a contraindication for this procedure. (C) Incorrect. An operative consent form is not required, but a consent form of some type may be indicated. (D) Incorrect. This test is noninvasive and does not require any recovery time. *Data Collection/Health Promotion (Thompson, McFarland, Hirsch, and Tucker, 1997, p. 1489)*

123. **(D)** Correct. The initial reaction by the person who has experienced rape trauma is often associated with shock and disbelief that it could happen to her, and a guilt feeling concerning how she may have brought the attack on herself. (A) Incorrect. The denial defense mechanism may occur but is less likely than the shock and guilt reaction. (B) and (C) Incorrect. These are not usual reactions to a rape trauma. *Data Collection/Psychosocial Integrity (Kalman and Waughfield, 1993, p. 321)*

124. **(A)** Correct. This is the only sized needle that would be appropriate. (B), (C), and (D) Incorrect. None of these would be a good selection for use. *Implementation/Safe Environment (Wong, 1997, p. 718)*

125. **(D)** Correct. A properly calibrated blood pressure cuff is essential for proper measurement. (A) Incorrect. A blood pressure cuff too narrow for the client's size will record an inaccurately high blood pressure. (B) Incorrect. The cuff should be wrapped firmly around the arm for an accurate reading. (C) Incorrect. This long period of cuff deflation will create an inaccurate reading. *Data Collection/Safe Environment (Perry and Potter, 1994, p. 225)*

126. **(A)** Correct. The proper distance is 6 inches so that the individual maximizes the safe and effective use of the walker. (B), (C), and (D) Incorrect. These distances are all too far for a

walker to be advanced with any degree of safety. *Implementation/Health Promotion (Ellis, Nowlis, and Bentz, 1996, p. 495)*

127. **(C)** Correct. This is a task that would be expected to be performed by the seventh month. If the 8 month old cannot sit without support, this may be suspicious of a developmental delay. (A), (B), and (D) Incorrect. These are more advanced activities than sitting and may be accomplished at different ages. *Evaluation/Psychosocial Integrity (Hamilton, 1991, p. 45)*

128. **(C)** Correct. By releasing check valves quickly, the client would drop too fast into the chair possibly injuring himself. Check valves should be released slowly to allow for time to safely guide the client into the back of the chair as the seat descends. (A) Incorrect. This is the appropriate manner to pump the hydraulic handle. Using slow, long, even strokes ensures safe support of the client during elevation off the bed. (B) Incorrect. It is correct to fold the client's arms over his or her chest, as this prevents injury to the arms during the procedure. (D) Incorrect. It is correct to have the support straps fastened securely prior to proceeding with the lift. *Implementation/Safe Environment (Perry and Potter, 1994, p. 826)*

129. **(D)** Correct. Epispadias is the misplacement of the end of the urethra on the shaft of the penis. The urethral orifice terminates on the dorsal surface of the penis. (A), (B), and (C) Incorrect. None of these are difficulties associated with this condition. *Implementation/Physiologic Integrity (Hamilton, 1991, p. 427 and Wong, 1997, p. 960)*

130. **(A)** Correct. The purpose of the continuous passive motion machine is to facilitate even healing of the tissue. (B) Incorrect. It is important to keep the leg extended without pillows under it when not in the CPM device. (C) Incorrect. The purpose of this device has nothing to do with the inoperative side. (D) Incorrect. The hip is kept in an abducted position after surgery, which is not true of the knee replacement. *Implementation/Physiologic Integrity (Christensen and Kockrow, 1994, p. 613)*

131. **(B)** Correct. This elevation, if found on three successive visits, would be consistent with hypertension. (A), (C), and (D) Incorrect. These findings would not be consistent with hypertension and fall within the normal adult range. *Planning/Physiologic Integrity (Christensen and Kockrow, 1994, p. 765)*

132. **(B)** Correct. For clients who may experience stomach upset, the best time to take iron replacement is during meal times. (A), (C), and (D) Incorrect. These times may cause additional stomach upset and can be a reason for noncompliance. Because a pregnant client may already be experiencing stomach upset, these could contribute to additional complaints. *Implementation/Health Promotion (Thompson, McFarland, Hirsch, and Tucker, 1997, p. 1247)*

133. **(A)** Correct. Immediately after the puncture, the first drop of blood should be wiped away, as it generally contains a large amount of serous fluid that can dilute the specimen and cause false results. (B) Incorrect. The droplet must be absorbed by the test pad to ensure proper chemical reaction. (C) Incorrect. Smearing causes inaccurate test results and should not be done. (D) Incorrect. Blood must be exposed to the test strip for a prescribed time to ensure proper results. The strip should lay flat so that blood does not pool on only one part of pad. *Evaluation/Physiologic Integrity (Christensen and Kockrow, 1994, p. 1105)*

134. **(A)** Correct. This question addresses the issue of an aura or predisposing indicator that a seizure is imminent. (B) Incorrect. Once the seizure occurs, an aura is not of any consequence, as the seizure is already occurring. (C) and (D) Incorrect. These are questions which

attempt to establish and collect information related as the seizure is occurring or after the seizure has occurred. *Data Collection/Physiologic Integrity (Christensen and Kockrow, 1995, p. 1117)*

135. **(D)** Correct. By positioning the client on the affected side, the strength and muscle stretching of the affected area will decrease the incidences of developing contractures. (A), (B), and (C) Incorrect. None of these are as effective in preventing contractures as placing the client on the affected side. *Implementation/Physiologic Integrity (Thompson, McFarland, Hirsch, and Tucker, 1997, p. 304)*

136. **(B)** Correct. An extremity that has not been used for a fluid replacement IV is best, as the circulation of it has not been impaired in any way. (A), (C), and (D) Incorrect. These would not be preferable to the arm that has not received any other intravenous infusions. *Planning/Physiologic Integrity (Scherer and Timby, 1995, p. 218)*

137. **(C)** Correct. It is necessary to actively listen to the client to obtain correct information. Once the data is collected and analyzed, the client's concerns and feelings can be addressed. (A) Incorrect. This would serve as a block to further conversation and would not do anything to decrease the anxiety. (B) Incorrect. Just because the client is upset and doesn't always make sense to you doesn't necessarily mean that he is confused. (D) Incorrect. This is too direct a statement and could result in the client's being intimidated and not answering any further questions. *Data Collection/Psychosocial Integrity (Kalman and Waughfield, 1993, pp. 1139–1141)*

138. **(B)** Correct. At this age the client is inquisitive and would like to participate and should be informed about the procedures. Providing a blood pressure cuff would satisfy the child's natural curiosity and provide a teaching/learning focus. (A), (C), and (D) Incorrect. These would not be as appropriate as providing a blood pressure cuff. *Implementation/Psychosocial Integrity (Shapiro, 1995, p. 476)*

139. **(A)** Correct. The most common complaint of a client with emphysema is shortness of breath that gets progressively worse as the disease advances. (B) Incorrect. Clients with chronic bronchitis (not emphysema) would report a productive cough, not a nonproductive cough. (C) Incorrect. Chronic lung disease clients usually have a weight loss and a decrease in appetite. (D) Incorrect. Chronic lung disease clients often nap for short periods throughout the day. *Data Collection/Physiologic Integrity (Thompson, McFarland, Hirsch, and Tucker, 1997, p. 151)*

140. **(B)** Correct. Too much magnesium will act as a laxative and is given as a laxative in the product known as milk of magnesia. (A) and (C) Incorrect. Both of these medications in excess dosages may cause constipation. (D) Incorrect. Simethicone does not routinely cause diarrhea or constipation. *Evaluation/Physiologic Integrity (Rosdahl, 1995, p. 1249)*

141. **(D)** Correct. This enema is made up of a solution which is 30 mL of magnesium, 60 mL of glycerin, and 90 mL of water. (A) Incorrect. A physiologic normal saline enema is safest for infants and children because of their predisposition to fluid imbalance. (B). Incorrect. A soap suds enema is most frequently used for cleansing the bowel prior to surgery. (C) Incorrect. An oil retention enema is an oil-based solution. It permits administration of small volume, which is absorbed by the stool. The absorption of the oil softens the stool for easier evacuation. *Implementation/Physiologic Integrity (Perry and Potter, 1994, p. 782)*

142. **(C)** Correct. Cheyne–Stokes respirations are noted in critically or terminally ill clients. (A) Incorrect. Dyspnea is defined as difficult breathing. (B) Incorrect. These respirations are defined as deep, rapid breathing and are seen in clients experiencing ketoacidosis. (D) Incor-

rect. This is a condition in which the client can breathe only when sitting up. *Data Collection/Physiologic Integrity (Perry and Potter, 1994, p. 158)*

143. **(D)** Correct. Kegel exercises are taught to increase pelvic floor muscle strength, promote circulation, facilitate healing, and improve or eliminate urinary incontinence known as stress incontinence. (A) Incorrect. This will not improve bowel function. (B) Incorrect. This does not have any impact on rectal prolapse, which will require surgical correction. (C) Incorrect. This is not a measure to prevent urinary tract infections. *Implementation/Health Promotion (Sherwen, Scoloveno, and Weingarten, 1991, p. 688)*

144. **(D)** Correct. "A nagging cough or hoarseness" is considered to be one of the seven early warning signs of cancer introduced by the American Cancer Society. (A) Incorrect. This may be associated with early lung cancer. (B) Incorrect. This may be associated with lung cancer. (C) Incorrect. This is a later sign of respiratory disorders such as tuberculosis or lung cancer. *Data Collection/Physiologic Integrity (Rosdahl, 1995, p. 1149)*

145. **(A)** Correct. The feeling that a person is somehow being punished indicates an exceedingly high level of stress and could be associated with resentment and an abuse potential. (B), (C), and (D) Incorrect. These are true statements that have no direct link to potential abuse. *Data Collection/Psychosocial Integrity (Kalman and Waughfield, 1993, p. 227)*

146. **(C)** Correct. This fits the description of a stage 3 pressure ulcer. (A) Incorrect. A stage 1 ulcer shows an area of pallor and mottling followed by erythema. (B) Incorrect. A stage 2 shows superficial epithelial damage which may range from a heel blister to as much as 4 mm of tissue loss over the buttocks. (D) Incorrect. A stage 4 ulcer reveals tissue destruction that extends through subcutaneous layers into the muscle and bone. The ulcer edge appears to "roll over" into the defect and is a tough fibrinous ring. *Data Collection/Physiologic Integrity (Rosdahl, 1995, p. 528)*

147. **(B)** Correct. Aphasia and inability to follow directions occurs as a result of damage to the Broca's and Wernicke's area of the brain, which is responsible for receiving and sending messages verbally. (A) Incorrect. They may present with this, but this is not as specific to a CVA. (C) Incorrect. The client with a left CVA will present with right-sided hemiplegia. (D) Incorrect. This is not directly related to a CVA. *Data Collection/Physiologic Integrity (Rosdahl, 1995, p. 1345)*

148. **(B)** Correct. Parkinson's disease is characterized by a shuffling of the feet without picking them up as they move across the floor. (A), (C), and (D) Incorrect. These gaits are associated with other problems such as CVAs or other neurologic diseases. *Data Collection/Physiologic Integrity (Rosdahl, 1995, p. 1034)*

149. **(B)** Correct. Crohn's disease creates episodes of diarrhea and abdominal pain. (A) Incorrect. Although this disorder causes gastrointestinal disturbances, it is usually associated with the lower GI tract. (C) Incorrect. Constipation is not a problem with this disorder, and medications are frequently given to decrease the frequency of stools. (D) Incorrect. Gastric bleeding is not associated with this condition. *Data Collection/Physiologic Integrity (Thompson, McFarland, Hirsch, and Tucker, 1997, p. 751)*

150. **(D)** Correct. Applesauce, although soft, is not considered liquid intake. (A), (B), and (C) Incorrect. These are included as liquids. Frozen substances, such as ice cream and ice chips, or semisolid foods, such as custards or gelatin, also are counted as liquid intake. *Implementation/Physiologic Integrity (Christensen and Kockrow, 1994, p. 732)*

151. (B) Correct. The proper position is to stand next to the client's affected side providing support at the waist so that the client's center of gravity remains midline. This position would impair his or her ability to use a cane or other supportive device at the same time. (A), (C), and (D) Incorrect. These are all appropriate measures to take when assisting the client with hemiplegia or hemiparesis to walk. *Implementation/Physiologic Integrity (Ellis, Nowlis, and Bentz, 1996, p. 493)*

152. (D) Correct. This position would provide the greatest degree of safety for preventing injury in a client with an exposed meninges and spinal cord. (A), (B), and (C) Incorrect. These positions would place the client at risk for permanent injury. *Implementation/Physiologic Integrity (Wong, 1997, p. 1173)*

153. (B) Correct. The seriousness of the intent may be partially judged by the actual plan described. The more detailed and specific, the more serious the intent. (A) Incorrect. Family support is important, but not as pressing as item B. (C) and (D) Incorrect. The reasons are important, but the intent is better assessed by knowing whether or not they have a plan. *Data Collection/Psychosocial Integrity (Bailey and Bailey, 1993, p. 235)*

154. (C) Correct. This is the proper method after urinating to prevent contamination with *Escherichia coli* from the rectal area. (A), (B), and (D) Incorrect. None of these have a direct relationship with, nor would they be a recommended intervention to decrease the incidence of, urinary tract infections. *Planning/Physiologic Integrity (Thompson, McFarland, Hirsch, and Tucker, 1997, p. 1159)*

155. (C) Correct. During the initial postpartum period, the nurse should meet the mother's needs and allow her to integrate the birthing experience. After this phase, she will then be more ready to take care of the newborn. (A) Incorrect. This is a process and not a phase of postpartum development. (B) and (D) Incorrect. These phases are not representative of the taking-in phase. *Planning/Health Promotion (Sherwen, Scoloveno, and Weingarten, 1995, p. 648)*

156. (C) Correct. A wedge-shaped pillow should hold the legs in an abducted position for 7 to 10 days postoperatively in order to prevent dislocation of the prosthesis. (A) Incorrect. The adducted position is the one that should be avoided, as this position may create a dislocated hip. (B) Incorrect. Traction is not appropriate for a client who has not had total hip replacement surgery. (D) Incorrect. When the client is turned, a pillow is placed between the legs in order to keep the legs abducted and reduce the risk of dislocating the prosthesis. *Implementation/Physiologic Integrity (Christensen and Kockrow, 1994, p. 613)*

157. (B) Correct. An allergy to shellfish would also indicate a possible allergy to the dye that may be used in the contrast of a CT. Any allergy to iodine would require the use of a different, much more expensive hypoallergenic dye. (A), (C), and (D) Incorrect. Any history of allergies would cue the nurse to especially ask about allergy to iodine in any study that uses a dye. *Data Collection/Health Promotion (Thompson, McFarland, Hirsch, and Tucker, 1997, p. 1489)*

158. (A) Correct. This is an excellent way to obtain additional information about whether the client is truly complaining about a specific problem, a general problem, or some other issue. (B) Incorrect. This response will make the client defensive and act as a communication block. (C) Incorrect. This is not a therapeutic response and would intimidate the client from continuing to explore the issues he is concerned with. (D) Incorrect. This would not be considered a therapeutic response. *Data Collection/Psychosocial Integrity (Bailey and Bailey, 1993, p. 130)*

159. (B) Correct. Lying prone after surgical correction of a cleft lip would not be recommended because the client could move his or her head up and down on the sheets and disrupt the surgical site and sutures. (A), (B), and (C) Incorrect. These are all positions which, when properly supported, are less likely to cause complications than lying in the prone position. *Implementation/Physiologic Integrity (Wong, 1997, p. 835)*

160. (A) Correct. In order to assist the client through the initial phases of the trauma, the nurse should work to create a relationship that is trusting and therapeutic. (B), (C) and (D) Incorrect. These are not considered therapeutic in establishing and treating a rape victim. *Evaluation/Psychosocial Integrity (Kalman and Waughfield, 1993, p. 321)*

161. (C) Correct. To be able to think about discharge and the short-term goals that will be addressed in the upcoming weeks, the client would ideally be able to discuss his plans for going home and further treatment. (A) Incorrect. This may not be done prior to discharge and is highly individualized depending on the client and the therapist. (B) Incorrect. To be able to fully identify strengths and weaknesses is impossible, as it is an ongoing process. Expressing anxieties may also take more time, as it is also an ongoing process. (D) Incorrect. This requires more insight than most clients have prior to discharge and should be considered as part of a continuing process. *Evaluation/Psychosocial Integrity (Bailey and Bailey, 1993, p. 223)*

162. (C) Correct. This is a significant drop in urine output and the initial assessment would be to check whether the Foley catheter was functional. (A) Incorrect. The physician may need to be notified after the equipment has been checked out. (B) Incorrect. Continued assessment only may place the client who is experiencing urinary failure or other problems at risk for further problems. (D) Incorrect. This intervention would not be routinely done in these circumstances. *Implementation/Physiologic Integrity (Perry and Potter, 1994, p. 739)*

163. (C) Correct. Discussing sexual thoughts at any age is considered normal and is not restricted to any specific age group. (A), (B), and (D) Incorrect. None of these would be appropriate to describe what the client is doing. *Data Collection/Psychosocial Integrity (Kalman and Waughfield, 1993, p. 339)*

164. (A) Correct. This medication works directly to stop hallucinations in a schizophrenic client and is also helpful in eliminating or minimizing paranoid ideation. (B), (C), and (D) Incorrect. The medication has no specific or direct relationship in eliminating these types of problems. *Implementation/Psychosocial Integrity (Bailey and Bailey, 1993, p. 144)*

165. (D) Correct. The use of sterile water will be least damaging to the newborn if he or she is suffering from any esophageal abnormalities. (A), (B), and (C) Incorrect. These solutions would not be used, as they may create further complications if the client has esophageal problems and aspirates. *Implementation/Safe Environment (Wong, 1997, p. 839)*

166. (C) Correct. Range of motion exercises will help prevent muscle contractures. (A), (B), and (D) Incorrect. These are all side benefits to providing for active and passive range of motion exercises, but they are not the primary goal. *Planning/Physiologic Integrity (Christensen and Kockrow, 1994, p. 274)*

167. (A) Correct. It is not necessary to wear caps, gowns, and masks when handling body surfaces soiled with blood or body fluids. (B), (C), and (D) Incorrect. All of the others are correct procedures to use within the guidelines of universal precautions. *Planning/Safe Environment (Christensen and Kockrow, 1994, p. 197)*

168. **(C)** Correct. The client who expresses this is usually trying to manipulate the nurse in a manner that will put one staff member up against another. (A) Incorrect. This is not what the client is attempting to do. (B) Incorrect. The client may be trying to create disorder and confusion, but it is accomplished through splitting. (D) Incorrect. This is a defense mechanism and is not an accurate description of what the client is doing. *Evaluation/Psychosocial Integrity (Bailey and Bailey, 1993, p. 101)*

169. **(B)** Correct. Obsession is defined as a persistent thought, and compulsion is defined as a ritualistic act performed in an effort to reduce anxiety. (A) Incorrect. This is not an accurate description of the client who is under an increasing level of stress, and a loss of contact with reality is not consistent with this disorder. (C) Incorrect. The use of neologisms or new words is not usually associated with this condition, but rather with schizophrenia. (D) Incorrect. This is not usually what is seen in a client under an increased level of stress who has obsessive–compulsive disorder. *Evaluation/Psychosocial Integrity (Bailey and Bailey, 1993, p. 73)*

170. **(C)** Correct. Cold, pale fingers are indicative of a circulation problem requiring immediate follow-up, as it is a limb-threatening sign. (A) Incorrect. This may simply indicate a normal finding. (B) Incorrect. Pain in the affected arm may be expected but would still require additional investigation. (D) Incorrect. As a result of the injury, the client may be cranky and irritable. *Evaluation/Physiologic Integrity (Wong, 1997, p. 1131)*

171. **(C)** Correct. Severe fluid volume deficit can result in altered thought processes, confusion, and restlessness. (A), (B), and (D) Incorrect. These items represent signs of fluid volume excess. *Data Collection/Physiologic Integrity (Scherer and Timby, 1995, p. 190)*

172. **(C)** Correct. This is the developmental stage in which the focus should be on establishing family and guiding the next generation. (A) Incorrect. The young adult is attempting to accomplish the task of developing an intimate relationship with another. (B) Incorrect. This occurs in the child during attempts to become more of an individual person. (D) Incorrect. This developmental stage is the stage of adolescence that helps to establish the role identity of the person. *Data Collection/Psychosocial Integrity (Freiberg, 1992, p. 338)*

173. **(C)** Correct. These areas should be washed every day, as they harbor the most microorganisms. (A) and (D) Incorrect. These would be included as a complete bed bath. (B) Incorrect. The axillary areas and the back must also be washed in a partial bed bath. *Implementation/Physiologic Integrity (Perry and Potter, 1994, p. 98)*

174. **(C)** Correct. When a nasogastric tube is inserted, a negative pressure is exerted, which removes secretions and gaseous substances and prevents abdominal distention. (A) Incorrect. This would usually be contraindicated after surgery until peristalsis returns. (B) Incorrect. This is not usually performed following surgery unless done to promote hemostasis for active bleeding or poisoning. (D) Incorrect. This should not be performed postoperatively until the patency has been established and the bowel sounds have returned. *Implementation/Physiologic Integrity (Perry and Potter, 1994, p. 952)*

175. **(B)** Correct. These symptoms and signs are all consistent with a toxemic state and need to be reported to the physician immediately. (A) Incorrect. This is not unexpected during pregnancy and does not indicate pathology. (C) Incorrect. This does not represent a toxic reaction. (D) Incorrect. Heartburn, indigestion, and vomiting in combination are not usually associated with toxemia. *Data Collection/Health Promotion (Sherwen, Scoloveno, and Weingarten, 1991, p. 923)*

176. **(B)** Correct. The left lateral position is the recommended position for insertion of a suppository. Lubrication reduces friction as suppository enters the rectal canal, and the lubricant used must be water soluble. The suppository must be placed against the rectal mucosa to facilitate absorption. (A), (C), and (D) Incorrect. None of these would be acceptable positions for administration of a rectal suppository. *Implementation/Physiologic Integrity (Perry and Potter, 1994, p. 537)*

177. **(D)** Correct. Obtaining vital signs is not a necessary step. Once the sterile field is set up and the dressing is in progress, the nurse may not leave the room to gather more equipment. (A), (B), and (C) Incorrect. These are all steps that must be carried out prior to removal of the dressing. *Implementation/Physiologic Integrity (Perry and Potter, 1994, p. 986)*

178. **(C)** Correct. The dressing must be free of all microorganisms and spores. (A), (B), and (D) Incorrect. These are not complete definitions of sterility. *Implementation/Safe Environment (Ellis, Nowlis, and Bentz, 1996, p. 19)*

179. **(B)** Correct. If the lesions are evident at the time of the delivery, it is recommended that the delivery be a cesarean. (A) Incorrect. This would not be an immediate concern. (C) Incorrect. This is not necessary. (D) Incorrect. This is a different disease. *Planning/Health Promotion (Shapiro, 1995, p. 148)*

180. **(B)** Correct. Clients who are prone to bleeding will not be allowed to use a regular toothbrush because the stiff bristles can cause bleeding. (A) Incorrect. This could cause bleeding if the razor causes a cut. (C). Incorrect. Rectal temperatures are contraindicated in thrombocytopenia. (D) Incorrect. Raw fruits and vegetables are not allowed because they may cause internal bleeding. *Implementation/Physiologic Integrity (Scherer and Timby, 1995, p. 159)*

181. **(D)** Correct. This test, also known as the ELISA test, is used in conjunction with the western blot in the diagnosis of AIDS. (A), (B), and (C) Incorrect. None of these tests are used in the diagnosis of AIDS. *Data Collection/Physiologic Integrity (Scherer and Timby, 1995, p. 498)*

182. **(B)** Correct. The person who has had chickenpox or varicella in the past have a definite predisposition to develop herpes-zoster. (A) Incorrect. This answer is not specific enough and less accurate than item B. (C) and (D) Incorrect. Neither of these have been associated with herpes zoster. *Data Collection/Implementation (Scherer and Timby, 1995, p. 1039)*

183. **(A)** Correct. This is the level of needs that must be met before any other level of achievement can occur. Maslow's hierarchy is a method of prioritizing care for many nurses. (B), (C), and (D) Incorrect. These are higher levels that cannot be achieved without first meeting the basic needs of food, shelter, air, and water. *Data Collection/Psychosocial Integrity (Scherer and Timby, 1995, p. 11)*

184. **(D)** Correct. The nurse is responsible for ensuring that the signature on the form is that of the person signing. The informed portion of the consent is a medical responsibility and is done by the physician or nurse practitioner. (A) and (C) Incorrect. It is not the responsibility of the nurse to determine this, as it is a medical responsibility. (B) Incorrect. This is not the reason the informed consent and permission forms are witnessed by the nurse. *Implementation/Safe Environment (Scherer and Timby, 1995, p. 239)*

185. (B) Correct. This type of infection is frequently seen in many clients who have impaired immune systems. This is also known as "thrush" and is a fungal infection. (A) Incorrect. This is the bruise-like appearance seen on the skin. (C) Incorrect. This infection occurs in the lungs and causes a pneumonia. (D) Incorrect. This is a tuberculosis infection that usually occurs in the respiratory tract. *Data Collection/Physiologic Integrity (Scherer and Timby, 1995, p. 133)*

186. (C) Correct. Checking for occult, or hidden, bleeding is important in any client taking an anticoagulant. (A) Incorrect. This would determine the level of immune system function or infections. (B) Incorrect. This test would determine lung and respiratory problems. (D) Incorrect. This test would determine possible problems with cardiac irregularities. *Planning/Physiologic Integrity (Ellis, Nowlis, and Bentz, 1996, p. 216)*

187. (A) Correct. The need to maintain clean lenses is important for safety concerns and for maintaining orientation to the environment. (B) Incorrect. This is important, but not absolutely necessary. (C) Incorrect. This information would have been obtained at the time of admission. (D) Incorrect. It is not advisable to perform a complete daily bath on an older adult, as it will cause increased drying and cracking of the skin. *Implementation/Physiologic Integrity (Ellis, Nowlis, and Bentz, 1996, p. 498)*

188. (A) Correct. The client on a low-residue diet can have vegetables and fruits, but they must be either strained or pureed to eliminate their fibrous content. (B) Incorrect. Hard-boiled eggs are allowed, but fried eggs are not. (C) Incorrect. Two cups of milk or the equivalent are allowed per day. (D) Incorrect. All whole-grain breads and cereals are contraindicated on a low-residue diet. *Planning/Physiologic Integrity (Rosdahl, 1995, p. 310)*

189. (B) Correct. Prune juice is high in potassium and would also help a person who is prone to constipation, such as an older adult with decreasing peristalsis. This would be a good recommendation. (A), (C), and (D) Incorrect. None of these are known for having a high potassium content. *Planning/Health Promotion (Rosdahl, 1995, p. 313)*

190. (D) Correct. The proper angle for an intradermal injection is 15 degrees. (A) Incorrect. This is the angle for an intramuscular injection. (B) Incorrect. This is the angle for a subcutaneous injection. (C) Incorrect. This angle is inappropriate. *Implementation/Physiologic Integrity (Rosdahl, 1995, p. 730)*

191. (B) Correct. The stools of the child with cystic fibrosis will be very loose and large, very foul smelling, and have a frothy appearance. (A), (C), and (D) Incorrect. These are not the type of stools to expect. *Evaluation/Physiologic Integrity (Wong, 1997, p. 788)*

192. (D) Correct. Mr. Martin is experiencing a panic attack, which is specifically characterized by the incoherent nature of his behavior. He is now in a fight-or-flight mode and needs intervention to reduce this level. (A) Incorrect. This level does not result in a loss of contact with reality. (B) Incorrect. This level is close to what Mr. Martin is experiencing, but he has lost contact with reality. (C) Incorrect. Tunnel vision is associated with moderate and severe levels of anxiety. *Evaluation/Psychosocial Integrity (Kalman and Waughfield, 1993, p. 82)*

193. (B) Correct. A sensitivity to eggs can create an anaphylactic reaction when given this vaccine. (A), (C), and (D) Incorrect. These are not contraindications to receiving the MMR vaccine and are not associated with reactions. *Data Collection/Health Promotion (Shapiro, 1995, p. 450)*

194. **(A)** Correct. The developmental milestones are a guide for the growth of the child, and each child may be slightly variable from these norms. (B) Incorrect. These are not a predictor of whether or not the child will grow. (C) Incorrect. The descriptions of developmental milestones are not vague. (D) Incorrect. These milestones were developed on extensive observation of children and infants and have been the object of a great deal of research. *Evaluation/Health Promotion (Neff and Spray, 1996, p. 280)*

195. **(C)** Correct. The National Academy of Sciences Institute of Medicine believes that this is the most appropriate amount of weight gain during pregnancy. (A), (B), and (D) Incorrect. These are not considered to be the correct amount of weight to gain. *Planning/Health Promotion (Shapiro, 1995, p. 104; Scherwen, Scoloveno, and Weingarten, 1991, p. 228)*

196. **(D)** Correct. This response decreases tension by acknowledging that the client may not want to have dinner, while reinforcing reality in a nonthreatening manner. (A) Incorrect. This statement is argumentative and will further agitate the client. (B) Incorrect. This does not address the agitation and rejects the client. (C) Incorrect. This is argumentative for the client and will not resolve the problem. *Implementation/Psychosocial Integrity (Wold, 1993, p. 261)*

197. **(D)** Correct. The initial plan should include the priority of adequate airway clearance. These other problems and diagnoses are also very important in this client, but they are not as pressing as adequate ventilation to prevent postoperative complications. (A), (B), and (C) Incorrect. These are all high priorities for recovery but less important than airway issues in the immediate postoperative recovery period. *Planning/Physiologic Integrity (Scherer and Timby, 1995, p. 866)*

198. **(B)** Correct. The wet dressing should always remain wet and should not be allowed to dry out completely. If it does, it must be removed and redressed. (A) Incorrect. The nursing or physician orders will dictate the frequency of changing the dressing. (C) Incorrect. Covering the wet dressing with a biologic dressing is not the recommended procedure and would impair tissue healing. (D) Incorrect. The solution for use in a wet dressing will vary according to the physician order. *Implementation/Physiologic Integrity (Scherer and Timby, 1995, p. 1033)*

199. **(A)** Correct. The proper way to initiate the wrapping of an above-the-knee amputation is to start at the waist and move down the leg and up to the waist in a figure-eight manner. (B) Incorrect. Anchoring to the thigh would create the possibility of the bandage falling off and not being effective. (C) Incorrect. This bandage would fall off, as it is too low a level to provide an effective support. (D) Incorrect. The client does not have a calf on the affected side. *Implementation/Physiologic Integrity (Scherer and Timby, 1995, p. 1009)*

200. **(C)** Correct. This is considered an open-ended question and allows the client to further comment on the requested information. (A) and (B) Incorrect. These are closed-ended questions that can be answered in a yes-or-no manner, without further elaboration. (D) Incorrect. This is a statement that does not require additional response from the client. *Planning/Health Promotion (Bailey and Bailey, 1993, p. 127)*

201. **(A)** Correct. The establishment of trust is essential to assist a person with depression. An open, trusting relationship must first be created. (B) Incorrect. The method of communication will be established on an ongoing basis. (C) Incorrect. This will take time and is not immediate in terms of goals. (D) Incorrect. The contacts are not aimed at making the client further depressed, but they may not relieve the depression easily. *Planning/Psychosocial Integrity (Kalman and Waughfield, 1993, p. 159)*

202. **(B)** Correct. The client needs eye protection while sleeping at night, and an eye shield will prevent accidental poking and damage to the operative site. (A) Incorrect. The client's head should be elevated 30 degrees to decrease intraocular pressure. (C) Incorrect. The client should avoid sleeping and positioning on the operative side. (D). Incorrect. Pain should not be an expected finding and should be reported immediately, as it may indicate infection or increased intraocular pressure. *Evaluation/Health Promotion (Thompson, McFarland, Hirsch, and Tucker, 1997, p. 584)*

203. **(C)** Correct. Constipation and straining at the stool may cause additional bleeding and other complications that are avoidable with stool softeners. (A), (B), and (D) Incorrect. These are not specifically indicated in this type of postoperative client. *Planning/Health Promotion (Scherer and Timby, 1995, p. 878)*

204. **(B)** Correct. The use of corticosteroids over long periods will create a cushingoid appearance for the client, resulting in the characteristic moon face, weight gain, and edema. (A), (C), and (D) Incorrect. All of these are not seen as a side effect related to the use of steroids. *Evaluation/Physiologic Integrity (Scherer and Timby, 1995, p. 791)*

205. **(C)** Correct. The cast should never be handled with the fingers or fingertips until it has completely dried. The palms will not leave imprints in the cast which may, after drying, create pressure areas. (A) Incorrect. The client will need some additional support. (B) Incorrect. Voiding time is variable, and the position may be different depending on the client's ability to tolerate the position. (D) Incorrect. The family should be taught how to perform neurovascular checks, but blood pressures and apical pulses are not required. *Implementation/Health Promotion (Anderson, 1997, p. 130)*

REFERENCES

Anderson D. *First Aid for the NCLEX-RN Computer Adaptive Test,* 2nd ed. Stamford, CT: Appleton & Lange, 1997.

Bailey D, Bailey D. *Therapeutic Approaches to the Care of the Mentally Ill,* 3rd ed. Philadelphia: F.A. Davis, 1993.

Beare P, Myers J. *Principles and Practice of Adult Health Nursing,* 2nd ed. St. Louis: Mosby, 1994.

Burrell L, Pless B, Gerlach M. *Adult Health Nursing,* 2nd ed. Stamford, CT: Appleton & Lange, 1997.

Chornick N, Yocum C, Jacobson J. *Job Analysis: Newly Licensed Practical/Vocational Nurses 1994.* Chicago: National Council of State Boards of Nursing, 1995.

Christensen B, Kockrow E. *Foundations of Nursing,* 2nd ed. St. Louis: Mosby, 1995.

Eckler J, Fair J. *Pharmacology Essentials.* Philadelphia: W.B. Saunders, 1996.

Ellis J, Nowlis E, Bentz P. *Modules for Basic Nursing Skills.* 6th ed. Philadelphia: J.B. Lippincott, 1996.

Fischbach F. *A Manual of Laboratory and Diagnostic Tests,* 5th ed. Philadelphia: J.B. Lippincott, 1992.

Freiberg K. *Human Development: A Life-Span Approach,* 4th ed. Boston: Jones and Barlett, 1992.

Hamilton P. *Basic Pediatric Nursing,* 6th ed. St. Louis: Mosby, 1990.

Kalman N, Waughfield C. *Mental Health Concepts,* 3rd ed. Albany, NY: Delmar Publishers, 1993.

Kane M, Colton D. *Job Analysis of Newly Licensed Practical/Vocational Nurses 1986–1987.* Chicago: National Council of State Boards of Nursing, 1988.

Kee J. *Laboratory and Diagnostic Tests and Nursing Implications,* 4th ed. Norwalk, CT: Appleton & Lange, 1995.

National Council of State Boards of Nursing, Inc. *NCLEX-PN: Test Plan for the National Council Licensure Examination for Practical Nurses Effective Date: October 1996.* Chicago: National Council of State Boards of Nursing, 1995.

Neff C, Spray M. *Introduction to Maternal and Child Health Nursing.* Philadelphia: J.B. Lippincott, 1996.

Perry A, Potter P. *Clinical Nursing Skills and Techniques,* 3rd ed. St. Louis: Mosby, 1994.

Rosdahl C. *Textbook of Basic Nursing,* 6th ed. Philadelphia: J.B. Lippincott, 1995.

Scherer J, Timby B. *Introductory Medical–Surgical Nursing,* 6th ed. Philadelphia: J.B. Lippincott, 1995.

Shapiro P. *Basic Maternal and Pediatric Nursing.* Albany, NY: Delmar, 1995.

Sherwen L, Scoloveno M, Weingarten C. *Nursing Care of the Child Bearing Family,* Norwalk, CT: Appleton & Lange, 1991.

Thompson J, McFarland G, Hirsch J, and Tucker S. *Mosby's Clinical Nursing,* 4th ed. St. Louis: Mosby, 1997.

Wilson B, Shannon M, Stang C. *Nurses Drug Guide 1998.* Stamford, CT: Appleton & Lange, 1998.

Wendt A, Clark S. *NCLEX-PN: National Council Guidelines for NCLEX-PN Item Writers Effective Date: October 1996.* Chicago: National Council of State Boards of Nursing, 1996.

Wold G. *Basic Geriatric Nursing.* St. Louis: Mosby, 1993.

Wong D. *Whaley & Wong's Essentials of Pediatric Nursing,* 5th ed. St Louis: Mosby, 1993.

Yocum C, Chornick N, Jacobson J. *Role Delineation Study: Nursing Activities Performed by Nurse Aids, Licensed Practical/Vocational Nurses, Registered Nurses, and Advanced Practice Registered Nurses.* Chicago: National Council of State Boards of Nursing, 1995.

Index

NAME _____

1. (A) (B) (C) (D)	30. (A) (B) (C) (D)	59. (A) (B) (C) (D)	88. (A) (B) (C) (D)
2. (A) (B) (C) (D)	31. (A) (B) (C) (D)	60. (A) (B) (C) (D)	89. (A) (B) (C) (D)
3. (A) (B) (C) (D)	32. (A) (B) (C) (D)	61. (A) (B) (C) (D)	90. (A) (B) (C) (D)
4. (A) (B) (C) (D)	33. (A) (B) (C) (D)	62. (A) (B) (C) (D)	91. (A) (B) (C) (D)
5. (A) (B) (C) (D)	34. (A) (B) (C) (D)	63. (A) (B) (C) (D)	92. (A) (B) (C) (D)
6. (A) (B) (C) (D)	35. (A) (B) (C) (D)	64. (A) (B) (C) (D)	93. (A) (B) (C) (D)
7. (A) (B) (C) (D)	36. (A) (B) (C) (D)	65. (A) (B) (C) (D)	94. (A) (B) (C) (D)
8. (A) (B) (C) (D)	37. (A) (B) (C) (D)	66. (A) (B) (C) (D)	95. (A) (B) (C) (D)
9. (A) (B) (C) (D)	38. (A) (B) (C) (D)	67. (A) (B) (C) (D)	96. (A) (B) (C) (D)
10. (A) (B) (C) (D)	39. (A) (B) (C) (D)	68. (A) (B) (C) (D)	97. (A) (B) (C) (D)
11. (A) (B) (C) (D)	40. (A) (B) (C) (D)	69. (A) (B) (C) (D)	98. (A) (B) (C) (D)
12. (A) (B) (C) (D)	41. (A) (B) (C) (D)	70. (A) (B) (C) (D)	99. (A) (B) (C) (D)
13. (A) (B) (C) (D)	42. (A) (B) (C) (D)	71. (A) (B) (C) (D)	100. (A) (B) (C) (D)
14. (A) (B) (C) (D)	43. (A) (B) (C) (D)	72. (A) (B) (C) (D)	101. (A) (B) (C) (D)
15. (A) (B) (C) (D)	44. (A) (B) (C) (D)	73. (A) (B) (C) (D)	102. (A) (B) (C) (D)
16. (A) (B) (C) (D)	45. (A) (B) (C) (D)	74. (A) (B) (C) (D)	103. (A) (B) (C) (D)
17. (A) (B) (C) (D)	46. (A) (B) (C) (D)	75. (A) (B) (C) (D)	104. (A) (B) (C) (D)
18. (A) (B) (C) (D)	47. (A) (B) (C) (D)	76. (A) (B) (C) (D)	105. (A) (B) (C) (D)
19. (A) (B) (C) (D)	48. (A) (B) (C) (D)	77. (A) (B) (C) (D)	106. (A) (B) (C) (D)
20. (A) (B) (C) (D)	49. (A) (B) (C) (D)	78. (A) (B) (C) (D)	107. (A) (B) (C) (D)
21. (A) (B) (C) (D)	50. (A) (B) (C) (D)	79. (A) (B) (C) (D)	108. (A) (B) (C) (D)
22. (A) (B) (C) (D)	51. (A) (B) (C) (D)	80. (A) (B) (C) (D)	109. (A) (B) (C) (D)
23. (A) (B) (C) (D)	52. (A) (B) (C) (D)	81. (A) (B) (C) (D)	110. (A) (B) (C) (D)
24. (A) (B) (C) (D)	53. (A) (B) (C) (D)	82. (A) (B) (C) (D)	111. (A) (B) (C) (D)
25. (A) (B) (C) (D)	54. (A) (B) (C) (D)	83. (A) (B) (C) (D)	112. (A) (B) (C) (D)
26. (A) (B) (C) (D)	55. (A) (B) (C) (D)	84. (A) (B) (C) (D)	113. (A) (B) (C) (D)
27. (A) (B) (C) (D)	56. (A) (B) (C) (D)	85. (A) (B) (C) (D)	114. (A) (B) (C) (D)
28. (A) (B) (C) (D)	57. (A) (B) (C) (D)	86. (A) (B) (C) (D)	115. (A) (B) (C) (D)
29. (A) (B) (C) (D)	58. (A) (B) (C) (D)	87. (A) (B) (C) (D)	116. (A) (B) (C) (D)

117. (A) (B) (C) (D)	140. (A) (B) (C) (D)	162. (A) (B) (C) (D)	184. (A) (B) (C) (D)
118. (A) (B) (C) (D)	141. (A) (B) (C) (D)	163. (A) (B) (C) (D)	185. (A) (B) (C) (D)
119. (A) (B) (C) (D)	142. (A) (B) (C) (D)	164. (A) (B) (C) (D)	186. (A) (B) (C) (D)
120. (A) (B) (C) (D)	143. (A) (B) (C) (D)	165. (A) (B) (C) (D)	187. (A) (B) (C) (D)
121. (A) (B) (C) (D)	144. (A) (B) (C) (D)	166. (A) (B) (C) (D)	188. (A) (B) (C) (D)
122. (A) (B) (C) (D)	145. (A) (B) (C) (D)	167. (A) (B) (C) (D)	189. (A) (B) (C) (D)
123. (A) (B) (C) (D)	146. (A) (B) (C) (D)	168. (A) (B) (C) (D)	190. (A) (B) (C) (D)
124. (A) (B) (C) (D)	147. (A) (B) (C) (D)	169. (A) (B) (C) (D)	191. (A) (B) (C) (D)
125. (A) (B) (C) (D)	148. (A) (B) (C) (D)	170. (A) (B) (C) (D)	192. (A) (B) (C) (D)
126. (A) (B) (C) (D)	149. (A) (B) (C) (D)	171. (A) (B) (C) (D)	193. (A) (B) (C) (D)
127. (A) (B) (C) (D)	150. (A) (B) (C) (D)	172. (A) (B) (C) (D)	194. (A) (B) (C) (D)
128. (A) (B) (C) (D)	151. (A) (B) (C) (D)	173. (A) (B) (C) (D)	195. (A) (B) (C) (D)
129. (A) (B) (C) (D)	152. (A) (B) (C) (D)	174. (A) (B) (C) (D)	196. (A) (B) (C) (D)
130. (A) (B) (C) (D)	153. (A) (B) (C) (D)	175. (A) (B) (C) (D)	197. (A) (B) (C) (D)
131. (A) (B) (C) (D)	154. (A) (B) (C) (D)	176. (A) (B) (C) (D)	198. (A) (B) (C) (D)
132. (A) (B) (C) (D)	155. (A) (B) (C) (D)	177. (A) (B) (C) (D)	199. (A) (B) (C) (D)
133. (A) (B) (C) (D)	156. (A) (B) (C) (D)	178. (A) (B) (C) (D)	200. (A) (B) (C) (D)
134. (A) (B) (C) (D)	157. (A) (B) (C) (D)	179. (A) (B) (C) (D)	201. (A) (B) (C) (D)
135. (A) (B) (C) (D)	158. (A) (B) (C) (D)	180. (A) (B) (C) (D)	202. (A) (B) (C) (D)
136. (A) (B) (C) (D)	159. (A) (B) (C) (D)	181. (A) (B) (C) (D)	203. (A) (B) (C) (D)
137. (A) (B) (C) (D)	160. (A) (B) (C) (D)	182. (A) (B) (C) (D)	204. (A) (B) (C) (D)
138. (A) (B) (C) (D)	161. (A) (B) (C) (D)	183. (A) (B) (C) (D)	205. (A) (B) (C) (D)
139. (A) (B) (C) (D)			

Other Nursing Titles of Interest

Review Questions for the NCLEX-PN CAT
Third Edition
Sandra F. Smith, RN, MS

1997, ISBN 0-8385-8445-4, A8445-7

Content Review for the NCLEX-PN CAT
Sixth Edition
Sandra F. Smith, RN, MS

1997, ISBN 0-8385-1516-9, A1516-2

ALSO OF INTEREST
Nurses Drug Guide 1998
Billie Ann Wilson, RN, PhD

Margaret T. Shannon, RN, PhD

Carolyn L. Stang, PharmD

ISBN 0-8385-7108-5, A7108-2

NEW TITLE!
Appleton & Lange's 1998 Drug Guide

ISBN 0-8385-0335-7, A0335-8

(more on reverse)

RN Titles

First Aid for the NCLEX-RN CAT
Second Edition

Donald L. Anderson, RN, EdD

1997, ISBN 0-8385-2600-4, A2600-3

Content Review for the NCLEX-RN CAT
Ninth Edition

Sandra F. Smith, RN, MS

1997, ISBN 0-8385-1507-X, A1507-1

Review Questions for the NCLEX-RN CAT
Eighth Edition

Sandra F. Smith, RN, MS

1996, ISBN 0-8385-8444-6, A8444-0

Appleton & Lange • PO Box 120041 • Stamford, CT 06912-0041

1-800-423-1359